Fatigue Free with Crohn's and Colitis

How Diet, Mindset and Lifestyle can increase your energy when living with IBD

By Greg Williams

Free Book Bonuses

As an extra special gift for checking out this book, I have put together some really useful free bonuses that will make turning your health around when living with IBD even easier and more enjoyable.

These completely free resources include further information on the foods to eat and avoid, a one page cheat sheet to follow each day to keep you on track to better health, and 2 fantastic tools to help improve your mood, positivity and mindset when living with Crohh's / Ulcerative Colitis.

Just visit this webpage now to get access
http://www.iamgregwilliams.com/book-bonuses-join/

Disclaimer of Liability

Greg Williams is not acting as a physician, psychotherapist nor a behavioural therapist and the scope of this book does not include treatment or diagnosis of specific illnesses or disorders. If you, the client, suspect you may have an ailment or illness that may require medical attention, then you are encouraged to consult with a licensed physician without delay. Only a licensed physician can prescribe drugs. Any mention of drugs in the course of this book should not be taken as medical advice. Any change in prescription of dosage is a decision the client makes with his or her physician. Nothing in this book should be taken as medical advice.

Rather than dealing with the treatment of disease, this book focuses on wellness, improved health and prevention of illness though the use of non-toxic, natural nutritional protocols and lifestyle advice to achieve optimal health. Greg Williams and this book primarily educates and motivates sufferers to assume more personal responsibility for their health by adopting a healthy attitude, lifestyle and diet. You always have the right to refuse any proposed ideas.

While people generally experience greater health and wellness as a result of embracing a healthier attitude, lifestyle and diet, Greg Williams does not promise or guarantee protection from future illness. You agree that by participating in physical exercise or training activities, and by following any nutritional, supplement and lifestyle advice, you do so entirely at your own risk. You agree that you are voluntarily participating in these activities and assume all risks of injury, illness, or death. You agree to cease taking all natural remedies upon the onset of any adverse effects, and notify your doctor immediately. You will also notify your doctor if you are or become pregnant or nursing as some supplements and dietary advice may be inappropriate during pregnancy and/or nursing.

CHAPTER ONE
Introduction

"I'm sorry but you have shingles"

They were the words from the doctor my wife, Donna, had gone to see when a rash appeared on her back overnight. Over the next few days, weeks and months the pain and fatigue was horrendous and worsened by the day. It was almost unbearable at times. She couldn't sleep. Every day was a struggle. This was the last thing she needed, things had already been really bad...

If we ever went away for the weekend, just walking around during the day would completely wipe her out. She had no energy for exercise or even just day to day life. The tiredness was constant. At times she was in tears. Anxious about leaving the house for fear of accidents. Living in fear of one day having to have a life changing operation. She was really struggling and we both felt like there wasn't anything that could be done. What little social life she did have completely dried up.

I could see how much she was suffering. We had spoken about having children several times but she definitely didn't feel healthy or energetic enough to do that. The shingles was yet another huge setback for her.

She had been diagnosed with Ulcerative Colitis 11 years before, when she was 20 years old. At the time she'd been studying for exams (which we think may have been one of the triggers for the disease). The diagnosis took forever. The doctors kept fobbing her off and just couldn't understand what was wrong. Her weight was drastically reducing and nobody seemed to know what to do. Things got so bad that she very nearly died.

Fortunately she was eventually diagnosed and given the medication necessary to get things a little more under control. The bowel movements (BMs) were still frequent and urgent, the pain severe, the fatigue debilitating, but she was able to slowly put weight back on.

Over the subsequent years this continued. There would be good periods of remission (although the fatigue was generally always present) followed by flares and hospitalisation. The advice she received from her consultants was minimal - limited really to medication and some pretty poor dietary advice ("eat lots of bread"). Through the years she was given several drugs, including steroids, which she hated. And now the doctor was basically telling her that the drugs they were giving her had suppressed her immune system so much that she was being left exposed to horrendous side effects, such as fatigue and ongoing risk of infections such as shingles.

My wife knew she couldn't live like this. It was at that moment, in the doctor's room, where she made a decision…

"If this is what it's doing to my body I am going to do everything I can to beat this fatigue, and get off of the medication forever."

That was it, it was decided. NOTHING was going to stop us. It was time to take things into our own hands. I literally became obsessed with learning all I could about IBD, chronic disease and holistic health and nutrition. Luckily I was already an experienced, successful nutritionist. However, I quickly realised that we couldn't do this through diet alone, and certainly not using the knowledge that the average (or even the best) nutritionists have. There was SO MUCH to it. We tried so many things (alongside all the drugs that the doctors were giving her). The vast majority of the treatments either made things worse, worked only in the short term, had terrible side effects or simply didn't have any effect whatsoever. They certainly didn't help with the fatigue. We realised the hard way that there were no magic pills.

Throughout this time I spent a huge amount of money on my education and countless number of hours with my head in books, journals, studies, and magazines about functional medicine, holistic health, acid reflux, IBD, Candida, parasites, the microbiome, nutrition and lots more.

Eventually after several years of endless amounts of work on a daily basis we finally had success. The system I developed – the one that helped Donna to transform her health and get to a place where she is symptom and medication free - is shared within this book.

Every day thousands and thousands of IBD sufferers across the world will be struggling just like my wife had to for many years. Struggling to get out of bed. Struggling to do all the things they want in life. Struggling to play with the kids, to have sex with their partner, to perform well in their job or in their chosen exercise, and much more. It doesn't have to be this way. You just need to be shown how, and this book will do that. We'll look at different systems of your body, move through an appropriate protocol and underpin everything we do using all elements of my own D.R.E.A.M.T. method and "5 Phase Thrive". We'll look at your diet, your sleep, your toxin exposure, your stress, your mindset and more, and by the end of the journey you can be feeling significantly better than what you likely do right now.

I honestly do believe that the information in this book is a perfect starting point for transforming your health and energy levels when living with IBD. However, as a thank you for placing your faith in this book I want to give you some extra bonuses to make the journey to better health as easy and enjoyable as possible. You can grab those here http://www.iamgregwilliams.com/book-bonuses-join/ .

Congratulations once again for taking action and checking out this book. Please keep me informed of all your successes, nothing makes me happier than knowing I have helped someone turn things around and they are now able to live the happy energetic life they dreamed of.

In good health,

Greg Williams

P.S. I know it can be tempting when you get something that you haven't invested a large amount of money in not take it as seriously as you would if you had invested thousands of pounds. Please don't make that mistake with this book. I have people pay me thousands of pounds for one of my programmes and I would urge you to treat the information within this book as if you had paid that sort of money to obtain it. Doing so will likely mean you'll take it more seriously, follow it more closely, and your health will benefit dramatically as a result.

CHAPTER TWO
Getting to the Root

A common problem for people with IBD, and the reason that so many suffer, so much, for so long, is that the doctor isn't looking deep enough to understand *why* their problems exist. Instead they are just trying to mask them. That's why I do what I do, and why I have helped many of my clients to get such great results. It's what the approach within this book will be aiming to give you an insight into. You don't deserve a lifetime of medication with horrendous side effects or life changing surgery when there is so much else that can be done.

Some people may perhaps feel that their symptoms are under control, or they may be going through a period of remission. However, even if your symptoms are reasonably "under control" yet you are using medication to do that, you could ask yourself if they are really under control at all. If you are requiring medication to keep things that way then all that's happening in your body is a constant fight between the medication and the underlying cause of the problem. Eventually the root cause ALWAYS wins and that results in more and more severe flares (and a need for stronger and stronger drugs, and possibly eventually surgery). And while all of this is going on, it's common for energy levels to continue to suffer, even if the bowel movements are under control.

Much of what is discussed in this book will be aligned with an area that is known as "functional medicine". It is completely different to a conventional medicine approach (which for me, is perfect for dealing with one off infections, broken limbs, emergencies, trauma, etc). As you'll no doubt be well aware, a conventional doctor will use drugs/medication to deal with problems/disease. This medication is generally designed to directly address the symptoms and essentially mask them.

You have an inflamed bowel? Here's some anti-inflammatory drugs.

Autoimmune condition? Here's something to dampen your immune system.

This approach isn't working with long term chronic conditions because the root cause of the problem isn't being addressed, and the overall health of the person isn't being considered. As you will have no doubt worked out, very few doctors or GI consultants are interested in a more natural approach to helping something such as IBD and especially have no clue how to help you increase energy levels / overcome fatigue.

I've worked with many people, helping them to get to a place where they feel significantly better (many symptom and medication free) following the protocols in this book. Yet even when presented with these cases / patients, many doctors still turn their nose up at what has been achieved. In fact, just before writing this I was chatting with a client who is now completely medication free, and in complete remission (and has been for over a year now). However, he recently had an appointment with his doctor who laughed at him because my client had told him he was managing his disease naturally and didn't need the medication that the doctor was recommending. LAUGHED at him!? Why the consultant even wanted to give him medication bearing in mind he feels better than ever, with no signs of inflammation and bundles of energy, is beyond me, but he could have at least been open minded to how it had been done, and pleased that his patient was now feeling so much better.

It's rare I will hear of a doctor or consultant who accepts that diet can even play a part, yet a recent study of IBD sufferers showed that many IBD patients in the UK do believe that diet affects their disease. Researchers at the University of Manchester developed a questionnaire that was completed by 400 patients. The results showed that around 48% felt diet could be the initiating factor in IBD and 57% felt it could trigger a flare. Worsening symptoms with certain foods was reported by 60%. About 66% deprived themselves of their favourite foods in order to prevent relapse and three-quarters said IBD affected their appetite, more so during a relapse. Yet despite all of this nearly half had NEVER received any formal dietary advice, even though two-thirds requested it!

Hopefully studies such as that will eventually make some doctors sit up and take notice and accept that people need more information, that their current methods aren't helping long term and are all too often leading to more severe flares and a need for life changing surgery.

So where the approach I will share in this book is different, and why it works so well is down to a few reasons. One reason is that it doesn't place too much attention on your symptoms. That might seem strange at first but a state of no symptoms does not indicate that someone is healthy. By masking your symptoms with drugs (or trying to mask them) all a doctor is trying to do is get you to a place of no symptoms. But that won't give you more energy. Or fewer colds. Or higher libido. Symptoms are the last thing to occur in a diseased process, and so understanding WHY they have appeared is important. Therefore, my approach places much less focus on the symptoms themselves, and rather identifies opportunities to build health in a person and address the underlying cause of their problems. It appreciates that when a body is healthy it will do its own healing.

To take this a step further, to be able to help someone with any chronic disease or illness, knowing the name of the disease/illness actually doesn't really help us. In fact, it only tells us what combination of symptoms we have, and then what drugs are commonly suggested for masking those symptoms.

Let's suppose someone was gluten intolerant yet had been consuming bread for most of her life. Over time this had contributed towards leaky gut (intestinal permeability), which means undigested food escapes through the gut lining into the bloodstream. The body treats this as an invader and calls upon the immune system to destroy it. Eventually this can weaken and alter the immune system and cause high levels of chronic inflammation through the body, including the intestines (side note - if you have IBD it is almost certain that you have a leaky gut, we'll talk more about that later on in the book). This chronic inflammation, combined with the appropriate genetic susceptibility, results in low energy, gut pain, frequent bowel movements, loss of appetite, loose stools, etc. So you go to the doctor, and following tests you are eventually diagnosed with Crohn's or Ulcerative Colitis. And you are given drugs. These drugs having been designed to address the symptoms (NOT the cause) of Crohn's or Ulcerative Colitis. I'm not saying that's necessarily a bad thing, but drugs should not be the long-term solution. The investigation is NOT over, in fact it's barely begun. WE STILL DON'T KNOW WHAT CAUSED THE PROBLEM IN THE FIRST PLACE!

In the example above, eating foods containing gluten was a major contributor towards someone getting IBD and its numerous symptoms. But it could have (dependent upon the individual's genes and many other factors) ultimately allowed antibodies to attack the thyroid, potentially causing Hashimoto's. It could have contributed towards arthritis, or depression or a whole host of other problems. You'd have ended up on different drugs, you'd have had a different name for your problems, and the symptoms would have been very different, but the CAUSE - the thing we need to identify to help fix you - is the SAME.

What does this mean?

It means that you cannot hope to be able to help someone into remission just by knowing the name given to their collection of symptoms. Instead, you must investigate the underlying cause(s) of their problems. In theory, you could treat someone with arthritis very similarly to how you would treat someone with IBD, and help rid both of their symptoms with exactly the same protocol (and conversely you could treat 2 people with IBD the same and achieve completely different results, because the cause of their IBD is completely different).

This is not an approach that most doctors will take with you, and it's certainly not an approach that the large pharmaceutical companies want you to take (a lifetime of drug use suits them just fine), but in my opinion, getting to the cause of the problem, and doing what we can to naturally improve the health of the person, is the answer.

Thomas Edison once said…

"The doctor of the future will give no medicine, but will instruct his patient in the care of the human frame, in diet and in the cause and prevention of disease."

That was over 100 years ago! For me he was right and this type of approach is the future of health, but it might take some time before the powers that be let us get there. Fortunately this book will show you how, while the rest of the world catches up. There is no better way to support what has been said so far than with a couple of examples…

<u>Surgery</u>
When someone has a chronically inflamed bowel, the

'solution' commonly taken by the doctors is to remove all or part of that person's bowel. Things can often get to the stage where that is unfortunately necessary. But its not a solution, and it would have perhaps been preventable if rather than just relying on medication up to that point, the doctor had instead looked at what could have been CAUSING that inflammation in the first place. Once identified, it could have been addressed, and the surgery could have very likely been avoided.

I have had so many people come to me after surgery, still feeling terrible, still fatigued, still with pain or bowel movement issues, because their underlying problems still haven't been addressed. The surgery / removing part of, or all of, the bowel, is essentially trying to remove a symptom, not the cause of the symptom. What's more, surgery can often makes the fatigue experienced by so many people with Crohn's or Ulcerative Colitis much worse.

Allow me to share with you some statistics around IBD:

"20-40% of UC sufferers, and 75% of Crohn's sufferers, will require surgery at some point."

Now that alone is pretty incredible and perhaps quite scary for some? The next stat though, for me, is even more so...

"50% of Crohn's sufferers that have surgery find the Crohn's has returned within 3 years."

That's pretty amazing, but unfortunately not surprising. You see, an inflamed bowel is one SYMPTOM of Crohn's and UC. It is NOT the underlying cause of the problem. Removing all or part of someone's bowel may give some temporary relief, but while the underlying problem is still there then the patient's health will never be where they need it to be to lead the life they want to lead. There will still be high levels of inflammation through their body and they will almost certainly still be feeling fatigued.

My wife is now so glad she never had to go down the surgery route and that we turned things around without her having to have a life changing operation, especially now she realises that it's not even necessarily the long term answer to feeling better. I fully appreciate that many people reading this will not be quite so fortunate as she was, but you will still find the information in this book of use, and everything will still apply.

Hopefully the above stats show you that the conventional approach just isn't working, and is unfortunately always about removing/masking symptoms rather than understanding their cause and building health. It is a system of "sickcare" rather than "healthcare".

The conventional approach works well for one off infections, broken limbs, emergencies, trauma etc., but often isn't, on its own, the long term solution for chronic health conditions. Don't get me wrong, I'm not saying that you need to ignore a doctor, or that surgery or medication is never necessary (quite often things get to the stage where it absolutely is) but it's NOT the solution that will get you feeling amazing, long term. Something else needs to be done to get you to that place.

With less focus on symptoms, a greater focus on health and appreciation that everyone is unique, coupled with an aim to find the root cause – amazing things can (and do) happen.

Ikaria
Ikaria is a small Greek Island that many people haven't even heard of but it tells us a huge amount about how to deal with Crohn's and Ulcerative Colitis. Its inhabitants live, on

average, 10 years longer than people in the rest of Western Europe and what's more, the people there very rarely suffer from the chronic diseases (such as IBD) now so common in the rest of the western world.

So what are they doing so differently to the rest of us?

Well firstly, their diet is almost entirely made up of nutrient dense, unprocessed foods. Fish, fruit and vegetables are eaten in abundance, olive oil and fish are the main sources of fat, and water, goat's milk, herbal tea and red wine are the drinks of choice.

Then there is the fresh air and outdoor lifestyle (the island is extremely hilly and the primary mode of transport is by foot).

There is a community feeling across the whole island. Friends and family are a priority. They work, play, socialise and laugh together.

Finally they sleep well, smoke rarely and often steal afternoon naps.

These factors are combining to allow a degree of health rarely seen elsewhere.

Now the lessons could stop there, and you could take this as a clear indicator that a more natural diet, less stress, more fresh air, activity, laughter and friendship will all combine to improve your wellbeing but there's an even more interesting thing to note…

You see, when an Ikarian leaves the island and decides to live elsewhere (a rare occurrence but it does happen) their health often deteriorates, and they are as susceptible to chronic illnesses and diseases (including Crohn's and Ulcerative

Colitis) as everyone else. Basically, when they are exposed to the same lifestyle, environment and diet as the rest of the western world then their bodies react the same as the rest of the western world.

What does that mean?

Well it means that Ikarian's are NOT blessed with better genes than the rest of us (so they aren't avoiding chronic diseases such as IBD because they have good genes). It is rather that the environment in which they live, the lifestyle they lead, and the nutrition they provide their bodies with are not allowing the disease susceptible genes to express themselves (you may want to read those last few lines again and share it with anyone who has ever told you that diet, lifestyle and environment can't possibly play a part in helping your IBD!).

This just goes to show that once you know you have Crohn's or Ulcerative Colitis, and once you get the advice you need to identify what it is in your lifestyle, diet and environment that is causing your problems, then you can eliminate them, increase your energy and transform your health, and you don't have to move to Ikaria to achieve it (though it sounds like it wouldn't be such a bad idea!).

CHAPTER THREE
Common Mistakes and Myths

Before we talk more about the Pillars of Health, my DREAMT principles and the "5 Phase Thrive", I thought it would be useful to first share with you some of the more common mistakes I see being made by people with IBD…

Thinking they are eating a healthy diet
The fact is that most people I speak to THINK they are eating a healthy diet, but really aren't. That's not their fault as there is a HUGE amount of poor advice out there in the media and coming from doctors especially. Healthy eating doesn't need to be complicated but at the same time, most people do need to be shown how to do it right.

In particular, your diet needs to be personalised towards YOU. Everyone is different and are at different stages of the journey. People have different sensitivities, intolerances and allergies. Some have UC, some have Crohn's. Some are constipated, some have diarrhoea (and therefore, need very different things in their diet). Some are underweight, some are overweight. I could go on forever, but suffice to say personalising towards you is critical.

It's also possible that people aren't giving the right diet enough time to take effect. While many of my clients notice big differences very quickly (there is often considerable changes in energy and bowel movement frequency in less than 6 weeks), not all people will experience such quick results. However, that doesn't mean they are doing things wrong. They just need to give it more time. Your body may have taken a long time to get to this point. And it may take a little longer to turn things around.

Thinking a healthy diet is enough

Eating a good healthy diet, that you have given time, and that has been personalised towards you, just isn't enough. This is why most nutritionists just aren't qualified or experienced enough to help with something like this. There are SO many more factors to take into account, many of which are covered by the D.R.E.A.M.T. principles and the 5 Phase Thrive.

Going for the wrong supplements at the wrong time

People place such a huge value on the use of supplements. In some ways they are right to do so as using certain (quality) supplements for a short period of time, at the right time, can provide HUGE benefits. However, most people are doing it wrong.

Firstly, their choice of product is often poor. There are a very limited number of things that will help you and most people are trying way more than they need. Secondly, their choice of brand is wrong. Quite often you get what you pay for and people are choosing the cheapest thing they can find or assume that if it can be bought from a shop on the high street then it must be OK (quite often it's the opposite!). You need to use specialist brands from specialist outlets. Finally, many people are just using things without really understanding why or without any real strategy.

Because of this I set up the Autoimmune Institute (www.AutoimmuneInstitute.com) which offers a range of very effective, pure, high quality supplements to people with chronic health conditions including Crohn's and Ulcerative Colits. I certainly don't pretend that supplements are the ONLY thing that is needed, but they can play a very important part so please do check out the website if you haven't yet done so.

Ignoring mindset

The importance of mindset should never be underestimated. In fact, I'd go as far to say it's the single most important factor in turning things around when living with IBD. In particular, truly believing you can turn your health around is so important.

Interestingly the majority (not all) of the drugs on the market show very little difference (if any) over and above the use of placebos. Especially long term. But people continue to use them (and believe they are experiencing results) because of the placebo effect. Surely this is a perfect example of the power of the mind.

Perhaps you feel you don't deserve better health? Or that you don't have what it takes? Or why should you be healthy when so many other people are still suffering? Beliefs like this can completely hold you back. Knowing that you ARE worth it, that you do deserve it, and that you can do it is vital to your success.

How you define yourself is also critical. Do you define yourself by your disease? If I asked who you are, would you mention your disease? Would you tell me you are a Crohn's or Colitis sufferer? If so, its worth remembering that's not who you are. You are not your Crohn's or UC, so stop defining yourself by it. Otherwise, taking action to turn things around will feel alien to you because it's in contradiction to who you believe yourself to be at your very core.

Finally, understanding your WHY is also vital. What's the main reason you want to get better? Can you see how it's affecting your life and those around you? How you can't play with your kids as much as you'd like? Or worried about your fertility? Or how your sex drive (or lack of) is affecting your relationship? Or how your career or performance at work / in your business is suffering? Getting in touch with the main reasons for why you want to turn things around can really help and lead to effective action.

CHAPTER FOUR
Pillars of Health

The root of problems within the body almost always lie within 4 of its main systems; the digestive system, blood glucose management system, detoxification and adrenal glands function.

I think of these systems as the "Pillars of Health". There is a high amount of inter-relation between them all (when the health of one is poor, this can have a knock on effect to the others). Once you establish a good base within these systems (underpinned by the DREAMT principles and my "5 Phase Thrive", both of which I'll discuss in a bit) you will find that seemingly unconnected issues will start to resolve themselves, many of your symptoms will magically go away, and energy levels will be much higher.

Everything I discuss in this book is aimed at improving the health of all these systems (which in turn will bring dramatic changes to your overall health).

Digestion
The main aim of the digestive system is to help break down the food that you eat and ultimately help to provide the body with the nutrients that it needs. The digestive tract is a vast area for processing and absorbing nutrients, and consists of the mouth, throat, stomach, small intestine, colon, etc.

The digestive tract is the biggest surface in the human body that has direct contact with the outside world. The function of the digestive system is absolutely critical. I'm sure this is of no surprise to someone with Crohn's or Ulcerative Colitis. However, it is important for all areas of health, even those seemingly not obviously related to the gut. For example, skin issues, brain fog, depression and fatigue all have links to poor digestive health.

If you have a poorly functioning digestive system you will struggle to reach and maintain long term health.

Blood Glucose Management

Blood glucose management is an area that a diabetic will obviously have problems with. However, if you aren't diabetic, it doesn't mean that blood sugar management is not a concern for you. Your body should very carefully regulate the amount of glucose in your bloodstream at any one time in order to help keep the body in balance (homeostasis). However, due to numerous factors (diet in particular) many people are suffering with poor blood glucose management, leading to numerous health problems. Fatigue, high levels of inflammation, light headedness, shakiness, poor memory, poor sleep, sweet cravings, frequent urination, and difficulty losing weight can all indicate blood glucose management issues.

Numerous foods can be responsible for increasing blood sugar levels. In particular, carbohydrates (such as sugar, rice, bread, potatoes, pasta) will have an impact, but also proteins and dairy. That's not to say that these foods need to be avoided by any means, we just need to control how much you eat, and when you eat them (which will be personalised to you and dependent upon a number of factors).

Adrenal Glands

Salt cravings, poor sleep, fatigue, tiredness upon waking, struggling to fall asleep in the evening, dizziness, light headedness when standing up quickly, large amounts of stress, and perspiring easily can all be indicative of adrenal problems.

The adrenal cortex is responsible for creating three different types of hormones that regulate mineral balance in the body, are responsible for increasing blood glucose levels, and regulating sex hormones (and, therefore, energy and libido).

There are several different factors that can affect adrenal health including poor blood sugar management, food sensitivities, poor sleep, underlying infections, bacterial issues and chronic stress. Essentially, the adrenal glands are only responding to what they are told to do. Thus, if you do have adrenal issues then further investigation may be required to find the root cause of the issue. An example of this would be if you have a bacterial infection in your gut that is putting a large amount of stress on the body. This would mean that the adrenals would elevate cortisol (stress hormone) in order to deal with the increased inflammation present, and over time, if not resolved, that could ultimately affect the functioning of the adrenal glands.

Detoxification
Our body is constantly being exposed to toxins from the air we breathe, the foods we eat, the products we put on our skin, the plastic we drink water from, and so on. Completely avoiding this toxin exposure is impossible and that means that our body needs to do a large amount of detoxifying on a daily basis. The liver is the primary organ within the body that is responsible for this, but if that is placed under so much strain that it is unable to function as well as possible, then that could mean that your body is not getting rid of these toxins as well as it needs to which could be compromising your health.

Hopefully you can see that the health of all of these systems (the "Pillars of Health") is going to be critical for your long-term wellbeing. To do that we will use the D.R.E.A.M.T. principles, and the "5 Phase Thrive".

CHAPTER FIVE
D.R.E.A.M.T.

Everything we do to improve the Pillars of health is underpinned by the D.R.E.A.M.T. principles which stands for Diet, Rest, Environment, Activity, Mindset and Testing. These things are at the base of everything we do. We will discuss these areas in more detail as we move through the book, but I will explain each briefly below:

Diet

Regardless of what the doctors may have told you, Diet is obviously very important. It is about nourishing your body as well as possible, and allowing it to heal, while ensuring that any foods to which you are sensitive, intolerant or allergic are removed from your diet. Food can either nourish and heal you, or add to the inflammation. Clearly, weighting your food intake to nourishing foods is going to be beneficial for your health.

As well as food and drink, we should also consider certain supplements that will help to get the body back to where it needs to be.

Rest

Quality rest is often an overlooked component in achieving optimal health, but it can have a HUGE effect. It is critical for both physical <u>and</u> emotional well-being.

One important part of sufficient rest is sleep. Studies have certainly shown that there are links between insufficient sleep and the onset of a flare in Crohn's and Ulcerative Colitis. If we don't allow our bodies to rest/sleep as much as it needs, then we cannot expect it to repair and perform at its best. This is a hugely important area that is often ignored, especially when it comes to beating fatigue.

Environment

Environment is split into two main categories; how stressful your environment is, and how toxic it is.

The impact of stress on our health and energy levels should never be underestimated. Almost all of the IBD sufferers I have known and worked with over the years have seen an increase in their symptoms when they are going through a period of stress. What's more, for the majority of them, if they have ever been able to identify a 'trigger' that they felt initially brought on the initial diagnosis of IBD, it was a stressful event or period in their life (exams, moving house, divorce, the death of a loved one, etc).

In terms of toxins, reducing the toxic load on the body can only be of help, as high levels of toxins (such as chemicals, parabens, mould, and heavy metals) will put a strain on the detoxification system (a Pillar of Health), and can lead to high levels of inflammation.

Activity

The types of activity you perform, and the amount you perform, can have either a beneficial or detrimental effect on your health and energy levels. Getting the balance right is very important.

Mindset

Mindset is a hugely undervalued part of your journey to better health, but it is probably the most important. There are many different facets to mindset but having a goal, truly believing you can achieve it, addressing any negative self-talk and not allowing yourself to be defined by your illness are all critical steps.

Because mindset is so important, and plays a role for the

whole of your journey, it's that which we will look at in the next section in more detail.

Testing

All of the above steps are obviously critical, but sometimes there are factors at play that things such as diet, stress management, sleep, etc on their own can't address. That's why we sometimes need to look deeper inside the body to better understand what is going on.

To do this there are a range of very advanced tests available to us. One that I very often run in a comprehensive stool test. You do this in the comfort of your own home, and it tells us so much about what is going on inside your gut (which is essentially the place where most problems start).

Amongst many other things it will tell us your good bacteria levels (which are really important for your health so if it's too low that's an issue), it will show any bad bacteria or bacterial infections, it can show if you have picked up a parasite (which is basically a bug), or have a yeast/Candida overgrowth. It can also show us things such as inflammation or how well you are digesting your foods.

Once these factors have been identified, appropriate steps can be taken to address the underlying problems. This will commonly involve the use of certain supplements. For example, if you have a parasite or bacterial infection (which many people do, unknowingly) then this can be a major driver of symptoms, and certain anti-parasitic or anti-bacterial supplements would be used to help kill off the infection (which almost always results in a significant improvement in symptoms).

These are tests which unfortunately a typical doctor doesn't run on his patients.

CHAPTER SIX
Mindset

Have you ever heard of Vilfredo Pareto? Perhaps not, but you may have heard of the thing for which he is most famous:

"The 80/20 principle"

Pareto developed this principle many years ago (he died in 1923), which basically says that in any system, roughly 80% of the effects come from around 20% of the causes. In his case, he found that 80% of the wealth was owned by just 20% of the people, but when it was looked into a little further it was found that the 80/20 rule applies everywhere...

80% of crime is caused by just 20% of the criminals.

80% of your profits come from just 20% of your sales.

80% of headaches come from 20% of your customers.

80% of all your results come from just 20% of your work.

(obviously it doesn't always work out at EXACTLY 80% / 20% but it's often pretty damn close).

This principle applies to our health too. I see so many people overwhelmed with where to start when trying to improve their health. They have a tendency to overthink things such as the latest superfood or medication. However, the one thing that will get you 80% of the results you are looking for is not a "superfood". The most important thing you must get right is your mindset.

Without the right mindset, then all other elements of the

DREAMT principles can be completely pointless.

What is Mindset?

In China and Japan, the number 4 is often considered unlucky, as the words for 'death' and 'four' are pronounced almost exactly the same way. This superstition is taken quite seriously. Many hospitals won't have a fourth floor, for example, and many people won't travel on the 4th day of the month.

This got David Phillips, a scientist, wondering about the effects of this superstition on people's health. He analysed the records of millions of people who had died, in America, over a 15 year period and compared the day of death of Chinese and Japanese Americans with white Americans over the same time period. What he found was really interesting….

In Chinese and Japanese Americans, chronic heart deaths increased by 13 percent on the 4th day of the month compared to any other day. The same data in White Americans showed no peaks on any day. Basically, it seems as though these people who were obviously very ill in the first place, and likely to die soon anyway, almost gave up the battle on the 4th of the month because of their superstitious beliefs.

Shows what a huge effect mindset has on your health doesn't it?

You can say that mindset is someone's attitude towards their health, work, relationships and just about any other area of their lives, and the core values by which they lead their lives. Our beliefs are created based on exposure to experiences, whether that be something we have experienced ourselves, or are told by people we respect or figures of authority. Even though consciously we may not remember everything that happened to us from day one, it is all stored deep in our subconscious and determines our outlook on our life and surroundings.

As an example, without even knowing, we may have a deep-rooted belief that we do not deserve better health and fulfilment in life. Or we may believe that we do not have time to look after ourselves, or that it is hard work to be healthy. If that's the case, then the good news is that all of this can be worked on. In fact, it is critical to work on it as, if not, the journey to better health will be almost impossible.

Goals / Belief / Action

To have the health and life you want, you need the following 3 things in alignment: Goals + Beliefs + Actions. Interestingly, when you have very clear goals and truly believe they can be achieved (the first two elements of that equation), then your actions will naturally follow and help to achieve that, i.e. it becomes self-fulfilling.

Goals

One of the most important things you must do to transform your health and increase your energy levels is to make sure you know what you are aiming for. If you don't know exactly where you're going and what it is that you're aiming to achieve, then it can be very hard to stay on track.

Imagine setting out on a long car journey to visit a friend. If you know where you are starting from, you HAVE to know where you are going in order to plan your route to get there. If you don't know where that person lives, how can you even start to plan that journey? You can't! But when you simply put the details in to your sat nav, your route is immediately planned out for you. Your brain works just like a personal sat nav. All you need to do is to find your destination, type in the details and believe you will get there.

Your journey to better health and more energy when living with IBD is just like that. Keep going with your main focus in mind, with a belief that you <u>will</u> get there, and you <u>will</u> get to where you want to go. There may be redirections here and there or an unexpected bump in the road, but keep going. Your brain, aka your personal sat nav, if it has the correct details and information, will get you to your destination.

So let's set our goals…

Setting goals is pretty easy to be honest. You just decide (yes 'decide', not 'hope' or 'want') what your life and health is going to be like, and put a date on it. The goals should feel realistic to you but be enough of a stretch to feel exciting and make you a little nervous. For most people reading this, I would suggest that a great goal for you would be to feel fitter and healthier and more energetic than you EVER have before, including in the time before you were diagnosed with IBD.

Imagine clearly in your mind what that would feel like, visualise the things you will do in life with that new body and energy. Imagine it every single day. Never lose sight of that goal. Make it your obsession.

You should also make sure you focus on what you do want, rather than what you don't want. Your goal shouldn't be "I don't want to feel in pain and fatigued any more" because that is talking about what you don't want. Instead it should be more along the lines of "I am fit, healthy and full of energy and can do everything I want in life". You are drawn to and attract what you focus on, whether that focus has negative or positive connotations.

Once you have your goal written down, carry it everywhere with you and read it at every opportunity, at least once a day. Maybe print it and put it on your desk at work. If you are ever feeling down, or feel like 'falling off the wagon' diet wise, have a read of that goal and remind yourself why you are doing what you are doing.

Over time you may find that your goal changes slightly. That's fine, you can refine and revise your goals all the time, but it's critical to always have a goal in mind.

Your Why

One thing that will keep you focused on your goal (and even help you to select your goal) is to focus on your why.

For my wife, it was the shingles. That was the straw that broke the camel's back for her. The fact her immune system had been weakened so much by the medication / immunosuppressants meant she had been exposed to this awful infection and the doctor told her that she would, more than likely, continue to be susceptible to this kind of thing for evermore. That would be no life and she knew there and then that we HAD to find a better way.

It scares her these days to think about where she would be right now if we hadn't put all of the work in to figure out how to overcome these problems. If anything, getting shingles sparked off our desire to do that. That's why I think it's important for you to answer an important question:

What's your WHY? WHY do you want to get healthy? WHY do you want more energy? Is it for your kids? Is it so you can have kids? Or so you can travel and see the world (without feeling shattered at the end of it)? Is it to improve your relationships with your loved ones? To boost your sex drive? Or give you the best possible chance at avoiding any side effects from the disease and medication? Perhaps you want to stop letting your family and friends down? Or be able to happily go out for social occasions without feeling anxious and exhausted? Or perform at your job or in a sport you love?

When you have your why, then no matter how hard this journey gets you will always stay on track towards your goals.

Belief
For years and years, people didn't believe that is was possible for a human to run a mile in less than 4 minutes. People had been trying, but failing, to do it for over a thousand years. In the 1940's, the mile record was pushed to 4:01 where it stood for 9 years. It gradually became accepted that the human body had reached its limit and it just wasn't physically possible to do it any quicker. Luckily Roger Bannister didn't believe such baloney, and on May 6, 1954, he broke the 4 minute mile. He had done what many thought was impossible…a super human feat!

Just 46 days later his record was broken.

And within 2 years, 37 people had broken the 4 minute mile!

It's not that a mile had become shorter. Or that training methods improved so much. Or that it just so happened there were 37 super human people all running around at the same time. Rather, it's that Bannister had shown them it was possible, and so they BELIEVED that it was possible for them to do it too.

What we believe is a very personal thing. What I believe may be different to what you believe based on our own experiences, how we were brought up or what we were taught to be 'true' at school. The real truth is you will believe anything if you can see enough proof and evidence to support it. Nobody believed the world was round until scientists proved it to be true.

Now that you have set your goal it is critical to truly believe that this goal can be achieved. If you have doubts, then it can adversely affect your actions. Tony Robbins once said that the "Holy Grail between someone taking action or not is certainty. If they are certain it will work, then they will do everything needed to make it work".

So how do we eliminate any doubts about our goals? How do we truly believe we can achieve them? Well, our experiences need to support it. Your experiences in life ultimately lead you to believe something. When you believe something to be true it affects your thoughts, and your thoughts affect your actions. Your actions will then affect your experiences and we are in a circle whereby we are effectively taking action that gives us experiences that justify our beliefs.

How does this relate to your IBD? Take this example…

Suppose you were diagnosed with IBD and the doctors pretty much told you that nothing, aside from long term medication and surgery, could help you. That's an experience (an unfortunately common one).

You believe it to be true (because you were told by a doctor, someone you trust and respect) and so your belief has been formed. Your thoughts are of hopelessness, especially when you flare. You take the drugs as prescribed and don't feel as if there is much else that can be done (because your belief is nothing can be done, because your experiences told you that).

And so, what actions do you take if you are having these thoughts? Do you, on a day to day basis, do whatever you can to help you feel better? Do you watch your diet, manage stress, avoid toxins, work on mindset, get the right amount of rest, sleep and activity, and test for underlying infections? No, of course you don't, because your thoughts, beliefs and experiences have all taught you that it's not worthwhile. So you don't eat well, you don't manage stress as well as you should, etc, and guess what? You never get healthy…which means that your actions have given you another experience that "proves" it can't be done, which confirms your beliefs.

A vicious circle huh?

Let's look at it differently. Let's suppose that your doctor instead said "I want you to know something can be done if you are committed. We might use some drugs right now to get things under control but for long term health I've seen many patients get incredible results when managing their Diet, Rest, Environment, Activity and Mindset, and Testing for underlying issues that we haven't identified yet". Perhaps he even gives you the names of some people to speak to who have done just that, so you can experience it for yourself.

That experience lets you BELIEVE something can be done. It gives you hope for the future. Your thoughts each day are about what you can do to build your health. They are focused on doing the best you can in all the areas that the doctor mentioned, and you feel that there is hope. And so you take the actions that you need to. You eat right, manage stress, and so on, and eventually feel better than ever.

The experience with your doctor gave you your belief, which affected your thoughts and drove your actions. The actions eventually helped to improve your health (a new, positive experience, which cements the beliefs created by the doctor).

Can you see how those 2 very different experiences have ultimately created 2 very different outcomes.

New Experiences

What if your experiences to date have led to a belief that you can't get healthy and can't achieve your goals? Are you beyond help? No of course not! But you do you need to do whatever you can to seek out new experiences and accept that your current held beliefs may not be true.

As an example, you could quite easily go online right now and find several success stories of IBD sufferers who have transformed their health using a natural approach (I have a success story page on my website – www.IamGregWilliams.com – dedicated to exactly this). But you could (if you really wanted to) go online and find people who say they have tried and failed to do that, and anyone who has managed it is just lucky.

If you didn't believe you could get healthy, you wouldn't go looking for people who have done it. You would only look for things that confirm your beliefs.

I'd encourage you to do it now. Go and find some examples of people who have improved their health naturally no matter how much in conflict with your current beliefs that may seem. Perhaps read through the stories and watch the videos on my website. It could change your beliefs (or cement existing ones even further) and that can only be of benefit in your journey to better health.

Blips

One thing to appreciate early on is that even though you have started the journey to better health, the road to long term success will almost certainly not be straightforward. There will be bumps along the way. There will be ups and downs, periods of feeling amazing followed by periods of feeling not so good. It's important to appreciate this fact in advance so that the down times don't affect your motivation and beliefs. If you give up at the first bump then you will never reach your ultimate goal.

Bearing this in mind, it's important to add the following word to your frequently used vocabulary…

"Blip"

From this day forward, if you experience a bad period whereby your symptoms return, you feel terrible, you flare, whatever, then you must just see that as a "Blip" rather than a "Crash" or a "Failure" or the "start of a flare".

"Oh, it's just a blip, I know I'll be better than ever soon enough"

Former US president Calvin Coolidge once said "If I had permitted my failures, or what seemed to me at the time a lack of success, to discourage me, I cannot see any way in which I would ever have made progress." Remember those words because they are so true and so important. You will experience problems, but they are just 'blips' on the road to success.

People
It is very important, as far as is possible, to only let positivity into your life.

There can be so much negativity all around us, and if we allow it to, it can throw us off track. For example, when trying to consistently eat the right way, people will tell you your food is boring, or say "Oh go on, just have some cake". Even though you know your food is not boring, and even though you don't really want a piece of cake, a comment such as that can lead you to make the wrong choices.

The fact is that some of those around us are naturally

negative people, and some naturally positive. It's important to cut the negatives out of your lives as much as possible. It's commonly said you are the average of the 5 people that you spend most of your time with. If any of those are the type to be negative, the type of person who doesn't have the desire to improve, who is happy with their dull existence, then they could easily be dragging you down.

Ask yourself if the people you interact with most on a day to day basis are action takers that get what you are going through, are supportive of you and who want to improve their lives (and the lives of those around them), or are they excuse makers, who moan and complain?

CHAPTER SEVEN
5 Phase Thrive

So now your mindset is clear, let's look at the '5 Phase Thrive' in more detail.

The '5 Phase Thrive' is ideal for people with Crohn's or Ulcerative Colitis. It is a structured, step by step approach to naturally turning your health around and increasing your energy levels when living with IBD.

It is perfect for helping to improve upon all of the Pillars of Health while utilising the D.R.E.A.M.T. principles. These are the 5 phases that my clients go through, and I assure you that if you follow these phases in the order given then by the end you can be feeling significantly better than you do right now.

CHAPTER EIGHT
Phase 1- Reset

The journey to a new you begins!

Our ultimate aim in phase 1 is to remove any stressors on the body. In particular, that will involve removing foods to which you are sensitive, intolerant or allergic to. Everyone is different, but this phase certainly addresses the most common problems that I see in IBD sufferers, and will effectively allow the body to 'reset', reduce inflammation and can dramatically improve your symptoms, sometimes very quickly.

Because this phase is about removing any stressors that are affecting the health of your body we don't *just* consider your diet. 'Stressors' cover a wide range of items but we must also place careful consideration on mental/emotional stress, any chemicals/toxins that could be problematic, causes of poor sleep (which is a HUGE stress on the body), and physical stress (perhaps due to excessive exercise). We'll do more on this in phase 3 but if there is anything big going on right now that is severely stressing you out, then addressing that sooner rather than later will be beneficial.

In this phase you should also conduct a complete assessment of your body, reviewing your history with IBD, your overall health history, your dietary history, activity levels, stress, metabolism, lifestyle, work commitments and goals. This could potentially highlight some information that you hadn't otherwise considered. One great tip to help with this is to write out a complete timeline of your life that includes any significant events, periods of antibiotics use, and health history. Doing this you can quite often identify when symptoms may have started, or when your health started to deteriorate and you may be able to tie this in to certain situations in your life. For example, many IBD sufferers will note that the onset of symptoms first began after/during a stressful event (such as exams, divorce, weddings, moving home, etc.). My wife first saw her symptoms when she was doing some exams. For these people especially this can be a sign that managing stress is going to be critical in helping them back to better health. Alternatively you may notice that your symptoms started after a holiday in which case that could tell us something else (quite often the chances of picking up things such as parasites and bad bacteria can be increased in certain countries).

What happens when we eat?

Before we get into the diet changes, it's worth understanding a little about what happens when we eat food.

The main purpose of the gastrointestinal tract is to breakdown the food that we eat, so that the nutrients from it can be absorbed and used by the body, with the rest being excreted (in a controlled way). The nutrients from the food allow us to thrive; they give us energy and help our bodies to perform to the best of its ability while protecting us against illness.

When we eat food, it passes from our mouth, down our oesophagus and into the stomach. Here it gets broken down further (hopefully it has been very well broken down already within your mouth, so take this as your first reminder to chew well, there will be a few more reminders to come!). Once partly broken down in the stomach it then moves through the small intestine, where it is broken down further and many of the nutrients from the food are absorbed. Any waste is then moved into the colon / large intestine which absorbs the liquid from this waste, with the rest being formed into stools and passed through the rectum and excreted from the body.

When someone suffers with IBD, some of these functions

are compromised because of the inflamed state of some (or all) of the GI tract. The breakdown of the food can be affected, the absorption of the nutrients can be affected, and the formation of stools can also be affected (which ultimately leads to the many symptoms of IBD, in particular fatigue and inconsistent, urgent, poorly formed bowel movements).

Understanding this process helps you to better understand the impact that the food we eat, and the way we eat it, can have on our health. We must help our body as much as possible in breaking down the food, so chewing is important (there's your second reminder already, more to come), and sufficient digestive enzymes and stomach acid are going to be important too, not to mention eating foods that provide us with nutrients and minimise inflammation.

Problematic Foods

At the start of your journey, it is beneficial to go through an introductory phase where you aim to remove anything from your diet (and lifestyle) that could be increasing the inflammation within your body. In particular you should aim to remove any foods that you are sensitive, intolerant or allergic towards, while at the same time ensuring your diet is as nutritious as possible. You would do this ideally for <u>at least</u> 30 days before moving to Phase 2. This phase might feel more restrictive than your on-going diet will likely need to be but it certainly doesn't need to be boring.

I appreciate it's not always easy to know what foods you do have problems with so below I'll talk about some of the more commonly problematic ones (which I do suggest removing from your diet for this phase). As we then get to phase 2 and reintroduce foods, you get a good idea of what foods are and are not a problem for you, which can stand you in great stead for the future.

Processed Foods

"I think it's all rubbish to be honest. Look at granddad, he has lived all these years, has never bothered with counting calories and all that stuff. He loves things like fry ups and butter".

That was a comment that my brother made at my Grandad's 90th birthday party when the conversation had come round to healthy eating. In some ways he was right - not about the fact "it's all rubbish" but about the foods my Grandad ate. You see, first things first, leading a healthy lifestyle does NOT mean counting calories and dieting (I'm pretty certain my Granddad never went on a 'diet' in all of his years!). Also, leading a healthy lifestyle also doesn't necessarily mean avoiding butter (trust me, it's almost certainly much better for you than margarine, though there may be some value in avoiding dairy for a while depending on individual intolerances and sensitivities), and whilst fry ups are probably far from 'perfect', I'd much prefer most people start the day with a nice amount of protein and fats rather than a bowl of sugar (Frosties, Coco Pops, etc). Again, it's only more recent generations that have decided that you have to start the day with heavily processed foods such as cereal or toast.

That's the main thing with the older generations; the foods they generally eat have always been unprocessed. I have hardly ever seen my Grandad eat anything that's been processed. Maybe the occasional chocolate at Christmas. Or a bit of ice cream on a summer's day. But it's pretty rare. Most meals consist of single ingredient foods. You certainly would never find him in McDonalds. You think he has eaten Turkey Twizzlers all his life? Crisps? Litres of coke every day? No way. Pure, unprocessed single ingredient foods.

If we just ate and lived a little more like our grandparents, the health benefits could be astronomical. For that reason the most important change that you can make in order to achieve great results is to keep your food intake simple and focus on unprocessed foods. Using single ingredient foods, perhaps to which you add herbs, spices, or healthy sauces means you are a long way there.

'Processed food' refers to food that has undergone at least one form of processing to turn the basic raw ingredients into the product that you consume. They will often contain poor ingredients which can do your body real harm. In particular they will often contain high levels of sugar and trans fats, and the processing of foods will often destroy a large amount of the vitamin and mineral content in the food, making it much less nutritious, as well as the enzymes, making it much harder for your body to digest appropriately. Essentially, avoiding processed foods means a focus on eating fresh, natural products without a long list of ingredients that you can't even read!

Known Problematic Foods
This probably goes without saying, but if you know that certain foods can give you problems then you should avoid them. Everyone is unique and the foods that do (and do not) work for YOU are unique. It literally could be anything. My wife, for example, found that she had problems for a while with courgette, asparagus and mushrooms. These foods aren't necessarily commonly an issue, but they were for her. If something makes you bloat, gives you reflux or gas or skin irritations or energy problems, then it's very likely an issue for you and removing would make sense.

Gluten and Wheat
I always suggest that the health of many people (especially those with Crohn's or Ulcerative Colitis) would benefit from a gluten free lifestyle, regardless of whether or not they test positive for coeliac disease.

Some people when hearing this would argue that that non-coeliac gluten sensitivity (NCGS) doesn't exist, and gluten is only a problem for coeliacs (and avoiding it certainly can't help someone with IBD). These people point to research (actually not "research", rather "interpretations of research") that suggest this to be true.   However, the primary study which many of these people use to support their argument does NOT actually disprove gluten sensitivity at all. It is a flawed study that is focused <u>solely</u> on IBS sufferers, and utilises dairy products in the diets of the participants (dairy is another commonly problematic food group and could certainly be skewing the results).

It's thought that around 1% of the population suffer with coeliac disease but my experience shows me that a far greater number than that are at least *sensitive* to gluten in some way, and many people do benefit from minimising it in their diet.

Is it actually wheat we should be worried about?
One argument often made is that it's actually wheat that is primarily the problem, not gluten. In the study mentioned above, when gluten is isolated it does not appear to have an effect (on very specific people) but wheat does. However, many other studies *have* shown that gluten is a problem (see below). For the general public, who just want to be healthy and feel amazing, a gluten free diet will still be cutting out wheat and provide you with the benefits you are after. But suffice to say at the start of your journey you will benefit from excluding wheat AND gluten.

What does the evidence really say?
The fact is that when we look at all of the research with an objective view point, it is clear that non-coeliac gluten sensitivity is very real. There are definite links, in various studies, to numerous conditions including autism, IBS, type 1

diabetes, skin conditions, schizophrenia, depression and allergies, to name just a few.

One randomized clinical trial that is certainly worth mentioning involved 61 adults who did not suffer with coeliac disease or wheat allergy, but who believed they reacted poorly to gluten intake. These were split into 2 groups; one group was given approx. 4.4g of gluten per day (in capsule form), and the other group were given a similar placebo capsule (that contained rice starch). After a week of taking these capsules each day, the participants switched into the other group. The researchers ultimately found that when the participants were in the first group (consuming the gluten capsule) then their symptoms (which included depression, foggy mind, abdominal bloating and intestinal symptoms) worsened significantly in comparison to the placebo group. Studies (and results) like that are very hard to argue with!

Real Life Evidence
Let's not ignore the real life evidence either. I have worked with a huge number of people – not just IBD sufferers – and barely any of them have failed to notice a benefit in how they feel from removing gluten and wheat from their food intake. That's not to say that they all now live a completely gluten and wheat free lifestyle 24/7 (many of them no longer have to), but they certainly felt better at first from removing it.

Are there any problems removing gluten from your diet?
I often say that "No one ever got ill from a gluten or wheat deficiency" and it's true! Rather than standing around arguing about whether cutting out gluten from your diet will be of benefit or not, why not just try it? Surely, if it helps you to overcome the awful symptoms of IBD then it will be worth it.

Many people unfortunately would disagree with the above. They, for some reason, suggest that a gluten free diet is not advisable and could result in a number of nutrient deficiencies. However, humans survived for a long time on this earth without gluten so it's quite frankly amazing that we are here today arguing over this subject, bearing in mind we lived for thousands of years without the very thing we apparently need to survive!

What do I need to be avoiding?

Gluten is found in wheat, rye, barley and any foods made with these grains. It is present in things such as bread, oats and pasta. However, it can also be in foods that you wouldn't expect, including some gravy, alcohol, dressings, and sauces.

A focus on unprocessed foods will obviously be beneficial here, but you should be extremely careful about eating out in restaurants due to cross contamination plus some of the oils, sauces and marinades that they will be using. That's not to say you should never eat out, you just need to be more cautious when doing so, and ask your server for their gluten free options.

Just one more thing to note here is that just because something is labelled as 'Gluten Free' that doesn't necessarily mean that it is 'healthy' or good for you. Food manufacturers seem to want to jump on the 'gluten free' bandwagon these days, and a lot of poor quality foods are being sold as 'gluten free' in an effort to entice the health conscious consumer. This is where coming back to a focus on unprocessed foods can be beneficial, as it can often be hard to even read the ingredients on many of these "gluten free" options (that would normally contain gluten).

Dairy

Intolerance to lactose (which is a sugar found in dairy) is the most common food intolerance there is. People who are lactose intolerant lack an enzyme (called Lactase) that breaks lactose down into a form in which it can be used effectively by the body. If you are, in any way, lactose intolerant, then removing dairy from your diet is hugely important. The chances of being Lactose intolerant can actually be higher if you suffer with IBD. If you have noticed problems after consuming dairy products in the past then this may well apply to you. Intolerance to casein protein (found in dairy products) is also very common (so you could still have a problem with dairy even if you aren't lactose intolerant).

Many people will eventually find that, even if they have a problem with one type of dairy food (cow's milk, for example), they will still be ok with many others (such as butter, cheese or goats milk). Dairy can be tasty and extremely nutritious so we don't want to exclude more than is absolutely necessary. Therefore, the reintroduction of dairy can be addressed in the next phase of this plan, but it's often worth excluding dairy completely during Phase 1.

It's worth knowing that a client, Becky, I was working with had no apparent digestive issues whatsoever but just suffered terribly with fatigue. Eventually, we identified that the cause of the fatigue was dairy, and as soon as it was excluded from her diet her energy levels increased dramatically. Just because a food doesn't give you obvious digestive problems, that doesn't necessarily mean it is ok for you or that it isn't a cause of your fatigue or other symptoms.

There are of course many other foods that can be an issue, but the above are certainly a great place to start. For even more information on the right diet to help overcome the fatigue of IBD, remember to visit this webpage for your completely free guide http://www.iamgregwilliams.com/book-bonuses-join/ .

Water

Ensuring that you are sufficiently hydrated is critical to your overall health and energy levels. Most reactions within our body won't take place without sufficient water, and the digestive tract actually utilises over 8 litres of water a day. Staying completely hydrated is particularly important for optimal energy levels. Obviously if the weather is warmer, you exercise a lot or have a particularly active lifestyle, then your fluid requirements will likely increase.

Supplements

Whilst supplements can be beneficial, it's important to remember that they are only supplements. There is no 'magic pill' and getting the rest of your nutrition on track (while sleeping well and keeping stress under control) is far more important than any supplement, so that should be your priority.

Having said that, some supplements can be extremely beneficial, at least for a short period of time to help get your body back to where it needs to be. Supplements fill 3 basic functions: Substitution, Stimulation and Support. They provide missing link between what is necessary for optimal health and what is missing from our food supply. They are often needed because it is impossible to obtain all necessary nutrients from food alone in today's world. These days the food quality is generally not what it used to be and does not have the micro or macro nutrient requirements to return the body to normal function from something as serious as IBD.

Different supplements can be needed for different people. They should be carefully chosen to reduce inflammation, heal the gut, improve the gut flora, increase energy, improve digestion, and provide your body with important vitamins and minerals to avoid any deficiencies that could be affecting your health. But we use them at very specific times. Using them all together can not only make thing confusing but it can hide underlying problems that we need to address through the journey.

There are a huge number of supplements available. Many on the market have no benefit or are of too poor a quality to be beneficial. This is why I started www.AutoimmuneInstitute.com where we offer very high quality, ultra-pure, effective supplements, designed for people with chronic health conditions. Please do check out the site and always feel free to contact our team with any questions you have as we fully appreciate that the world of supplements can be a very confusing area. The products I recommend below are offered by Autoimmune Institute but please know that I am only recommending them because I have seen the results they can achieve and know how beneficial they can be. I certainly don't ever pretend that supplements are magic pills, or the only thing needed, but the right ones, at the right time, can help.

Sequencing and Titration

When beginning a supplementation regime, or when introducing new supplements, it is prudent to take a "sequencing and titration" approach.

'Titration' is whereby you will gradually increase the dosage of the supplement over a period of time. For example, you might start by taking one drop of a certain supplement, and increase this dosage by 1 drop each time, up to a specified maximum (assuming there is no reaction in the meantime). If a certain dosage does create an adverse reaction, then the dosage can be reduced to previous level where no negatives occurred and it can be maintained at that level. This obviously helps to identify the appropriate dosage for each person.

'Sequencing' is when you start using just one product at a time, rather than start using multiple supplements at the same time. In particular, this approach helps to identify any adverse reactions to a specific product.

Sequencing and titration therefore help to improve your results while minimising or eliminating adverse reactions

Phase 1 Supplements
Below are some supplements that you may want to consider introducing towards the start of the "5 Phase Thrive".

Please ensure you follow the instructions on the label of any supplements you use and consult your physician before taking anything. Also, it is your responsibility to read the label and check for any ingredients that you may find problematic.

Turmeric
Turmeric has numerous benefits and, in particular, can help to support the inflammatory response in the body as well as digestive health. Considering that inflammation is the main cause of symptoms in someone with IBD then a good quality turmeric supplement can be extremely beneficial.

Inflammation is also a major cause of a vitamin B12 deficiency (which many IBD sufferers experience). This is because B12 is primarily absorbed through the small intestine, so when that is inflamed, then B12 won't be absorbed as effectively. B12 is critical for energy levels, making this one of the main drivers of fatigue in someone with Crohn's or Ulcerative Colitis. However, simply relying on B12 supplements or injections often isn't as effective as it should be because without addressing the inflammation, then it will still not be absorbed as well as is needed. That's why supplements for inflammation, and the rest of the strategies in this book, can be so important, and help energy levels so much,

The Advanced Turmeric from the Autoimmune Institute contains organic turmeric (and so helps to avoid the toxins often found in non-organic turmeric), and is mixed with Bioperine, a black pepper extract, which improves the absorption of the beneficial factors within turmeric. Visit www.AutoimmuneInstitute.com/advancedturmeric for more information.

Omega 3 (Fish Oil)
Omega 3 / Fish Oils are really important for overall health and, in particular, have been shown to have anti-inflammatory benefits. Additionally they help with things such as fat loss, improved insulin sensitivity, improved skin condition, and much more.

If you are eating oily fish (salmon, mackerel, sardines) at least three times a week, then supplemental fish oil probably isn't all that essential and you can save your money, but otherwise it can be a really useful addition. Check out the "Advanced Fish Oil" at www.AutoimmuneInstitute.com for a very high quality, pure, high strength fish oil.

Proibiotics
Our guts are home to millions of different types of bacteria. These are critical for everyone's health and impact pretty much everything including energy, bowel movements, inflammation, skin condition, pain, mood, allergies, digestion, emotions and more.

However, things such as medication, antibiotics, travel, stress, diet and toxin exposure can disrupt the bacteria in the gut, and this can lead to many symptoms.

Probiotics are 'good' or 'friendly' bacteria that can help to improve the balance of bacteria within us, and so can often have various health benefits.

They can also help to fight problem bacteria, parasites, and candida overgrowth that so many people are (often unknowingly) suffering with and which cause major symptoms in people with chronic health conditions.

Probiotics are often found in supplements, as well as certain foods and yoghurts.

From a food perspective, fermented foods such as kefir, sauerkraut, and kimchi can all be good sources of beneficial bacteria. Some of these can be made at home, but it's normally much easier to buy online or from a good quality health food store.

With regard to the yoghurts and drinks that are found in many supermarkets these are, unfortunately, for most people, completely useless. That's because they are filled with sugar, and by the time the supposedly beneficial live bacteria reach your gut, they are completely dead and, therefore, ineffective.

This is why supplements can be so beneficial. However, if you do take a supplement, the quality of that supplement is very important. In particular, the delivery of it and how much beneficial live bacteria actually reaches your gut is essential for you to derive the benefits from it. Unfortunately, there are very few on the market with sufficient quantities of bacteria in in the first place, or sufficiently designed to survive transit through the body, which is why it can be so easy to waste money.

The fact is that probiotics will work for some people, and not for others. And certain brands of probiotics supplements will work some people, and another brand will work for others. This is because we are all different and need different things. Different probiotics provide different strains and amounts of bacteria, which we will all react differently to. Therefore, some experimentation and time can sometimes be needed.

At the Autoimmune Institute, we offer 2 different types of probiotic. The first is "Advanced Flora". This is a high strength (20bn CFU) probiotic that has an innovative capsule that ensures the bacteria survive as they pass through the acid in the stomach (this is a problem with most other probiotics). It provides the body with 6 of the most beneficial known bacterial strains.

The other product is "Advanced Protection". This contains a probiotic yeast known as Saccharomyces Boulardii that has been shown to have a huge number of benefits for people with Crohn's and Colitis, or people suffering from Clostridium Difficile or Antibiotic Associated Diarrhoea.

It's also often really beneficial for people who are travelling abroad (when you are more likely to pick up bugs/infections), when you have diarrhoea or when you need to take antibiotics.

Multi Vitamin / Vitamin D

Taking a multi vitamin can help to ensure that you are getting all the nutrients you need into your body. Ideally we would get all of our required nutrients from our food but this isn't always possible, meaning many people are deficient in one or more vitamins (perhaps without realising it), and a quality multi vitamin can help to resolve this and be a good insurance policy.

In particular, adequate levels of Vitamin D are extremely important. The majority of people, unless they work outside during the day in a sunny climate, will be deficient in vitamin D. Adequate vitamin D levels can aid a strong immune system, assist fat loss, increase free testosterone, and support bone health. It can play a role in reducing the risk of certain cancers, as well as diabetes. There certainly appears to be a link between vitamin D deficiency and incidents of autoimmune conditions such as Crohn's and Ulcerative Colitis.

Vitamin D testing is relatively cheap, so it can be worth testing your levels a few times a year to make sure they are adequate. You can then adjust your supplemental use accordingly. You can arrange for those tests through my website.

People who suffer with IBD and who are in an inflamed state do have an increased risk of certain vitamin deficiencies. This is for various reasons but blood loss and poor absorption in the small intestine are the primary causes. Obviously any surgery/removal of the small intestine will too have an impact. Iron and B12 deficiency can be especially common (your doctor should be able to test for this and advise appropriately). This can be a major cause of fatigue. For this reason, supplementation with a good quality multi vitamin may be worthwhile but it should not be the only solution and increasing iron and B vitamin intake through the diet (red meat, eggs, green vegetables in particular) should also be considered, while obviously working on reducing the inflammation levels to help improve absorption (this is where things such as turmeric and fish oil can be beneficial as they have been shown to potentially have anti-inflammatory properties).

I don't consider a multi vitamin to be an essential supplement, but vitamin D almost always is. Also, I don't recommend supplementation of iron unless your doctor has tested your levels and specifically advised it to be necessary.

Testing

Inflammatory Bowel Disease is obviously very serious and complicated, and while the diet, lifestyle changes, and the specific phases we go through in this book can help to dramatically turn around your health, something that can be a fantastic additional tool for helping us better understand what's going on inside your body is some functional lab testing. There are a range of really advanced tests available to you, the majority of which most other IBD sufferers do not even know about. They allow us to further personalise the programme towards you and give us the best possible chance at further improving your health, energy levels, digestive issues and reducing your pain.

I like to think of these tests as a way to "look under the hood" and truly understand what's going on inside the body..

The list of available tests is huge but includes the ability to check for the presence of parasites, yeast growth, imbalanced gut bacteria, liver function, adrenal function, food sensitivities and much more. All these things can severely impact your health and chances of success. Once the test results are back, they can be analysed and personalised protocols will then be put in place, if necessary

Functional testing differs from conventional testing that a doctor may have done with you in a couple of ways. Primarily, the tests that I would use with my private clients would be performed by specialist laboratories who use very advanced methods to look into and analyse the samples provided. All too often I have seen tests done by a GP show nothing wrong, but when we run our tests we almost always uncover things that need to be addressed. If done correctly these tests should not be used to diagnose disease but rather look for opportunities to heal and improve health in your body.

I believe that everyone would benefit from testing but especially those people who are already closely following the advice in this book but haven't noticed significant health changes, or those people who are willing to do whatever it takes to transform their health and want quick results.

If you feel you are at the stage where some lab testing is required, then please contact my team through my website and we can arrange a time to discuss your options.

Here are some of the most beneficial tests that you can do:

Stool Test
This is a comprehensive stool test (done at home) that checks for the presence of pathogens such as parasites, and bacterial imbalances as well as digestive function. These can be very common in an IBD sufferer because of the weakened immune system and addressing them is absolutely critical as they can wreak havoc on your digestive system.

The test is a 3 day stool test (meaning samples are taken over a 3 day period). This is because pathogens can very easily be missed when using just one sample. Additionally, the labs who assess the samples use extremely advanced methods to identify if there is anything within your stool that shouldn't be there. Your doctor may have given you a stool test in the past but it was almost certainly a one day test that uses relatively poor testing methodologies to assess the results (and, therefore, would have very likely missed things of importance).

Suppose your timeline showed you that your symptoms significantly worsened after a holiday abroad. In these cases, this can quite often tie in with the fact you picked up a parasite, or some kind of infection, bacteria, etc (as it can often be easier to pick up this type of thing in certain countries). If that's the case then a comprehensive stool test can certainly be worthwhile.

For someone with digestive health issues, I believe a stool test to almost always be the single most important test that you can first do.

Organic Acid Test

This simple urine test looks at a huge range of markers and in particular, can indicate intestinal yeast and bacterial problems, as well as nutrient deficiencies. Abnormally high levels of these microorganisms can cause or worsen behaviour disorders, hyperactivity, movement disorders, fatigue and immune function. Many people with chronic illnesses (such as IBD) and neurological disorders often excrete several abnormal organic acids. If abnormalities are detected then appropriate protocols can be put in place to address them.

Adrenal Stress Indicator

This is a saliva test that can be done at home. 4 Saliva samples are taken through the day which allows us to measure the effectiveness of your adrenal glands and check for steroid hormone imbalances, both of which are critical for overall health, especially energy. The test itself takes markers for a number of important hormones including cortisol (a very important hormone for energy), progesterone, testosterone, DHEA, and oestrogen. As well as giving us a much greater insight into energy levels, sex drive and muscle building/fat burning ability, this can be a really important test for women who suffer with PMT.

Vitamin D

Vitamin D deficiency is a huge problem in the world today and is heavily linked with autoimmune conditions such as Crohn's and Ulcerative Colitis. This test, which requires a simple finger prick blood test, done at home, can quickly highlight if you have a deficiency, and to what extent, which will allow us to take appropriate action. I personally use this relatively inexpensive test twice a year to check my levels, which allows me to supplement appropriately.

Parasites / Bacteria

I've been to Thailand a couple of times; once on my

honeymoon and then again for a friend's wedding. Both times I absolutely fell in love with the place - the vibe, the people, the food. Everything was truly amazing. However, both times we have been my wife has been very ill. Before the last time we went she had felt the best she had been in years and years. We'd already addressed a lot with her diet and lifestyle and it made a huge difference; she was full of energy, the bowel movements (BM's) were under control and there was no sign of her UC at all. That quickly changed though on holiday, when she suddenly started to get ill (despite relaxing and continuing to eat well). The BM's, in particular, increased in frequency and urgency, and this continued for a long time, even once we were home. After lots of trial and error, and some testing, we identified that she had picked up a parasite which we were able to kill off using an appropriate protocol and her health quickly returned.

This showed me the effect that things like parasites can have on someone's health, even when everything else is being done incredibly well. Therefore, I wanted to share more information on this area in case you are scratching your head about what is causing your on-going symptoms. The thought of having a parasite or bacterial infection inside you is probably pretty scary, but they are actually much more common than you might realise.

What is a parasite?
A parasite is basically anything that survives by feeding off of another organism. The parasites that I'm referring to here are basically small bugs/worms that live in your digestion system and will feed off of you and your food intake. They are dependent upon you to survive. There are a huge number of different types of parasite that will cause a range of symptoms (and will affect different people in different ways).

How do you get parasites?

While in my wife's case she seemed to pick hers up in Thailand (which is very commonly done) it's not true that you can only pick them up in under-developed countries. You can get them absolutely anywhere so don't rule out the possibility that you have one just because you haven't travelled much. I once found 7 different types of parasite in a client who had never left the UK!

They will generally get into the body through food and water. Unclean or undercooked food can be a common way that you will contract a parasite or bacterial infection, as is swimming in lakes and rivers. It is also possible to be passed a infection from an animal or another human (especially if their hygiene is not as good as it should be - washing hands regularly for example).

How do I know if I have a parasite or bacterial infection?
The best way to check is using a good quality stool test. A doctor may have already run one of these on you but, as already explained, due to the accuracy of the testing they typically use, the parasite could have easily been missed.

What do you do if you have one?
There are a range of alternatives that you will have available to you to kill off the infection. I'm obliged to advise that you should always consult your GP should you find that you have one, and they may prescribe antibiotics to help with that. However, if you understandably didn't want to go down that route, a more natural approach is also often possible. The required protocol will be determined on a case by case basis and, in particular, will need to consider the person and the infections that they have.

Yeast / Candida
As well as paraistes and bacterial infections, yeast or

Candida overgrowth is another very common problem that I see that can be a major driver of symptoms in someone with Crohn's or Ulcerative Colitis, including bloating, infections, skin problems, mood swings, fatigue, brain fog, digestive issues, extreme sweet cravings and much more.

What is Candida?
Candida is a type of yeast or fungus. Everyone has small amounts of Candida within their mouth and intestines, and in small amounts, it can be helpful in aiding digestion and nutrient absorption. However, when it overgrows it becomes a problem, making its way into the bloodstream and releasing toxins into the body. This leads to numerous symptoms as the body attempts to fight it off.

How do you get a Candida overgrowth?
Candida is opportunistic in that it overgrows because it is allowed to. This happens when conditions in the gut aren't as good as they could be.

The good bacteria in the gut plays an important role in preventing Candida overgrowth. With low levels of good bacteria someone will be much more exposed to the possibility of Candida overgrowth. Levels of good bacteria are affected by many things including stress, poor diet, medication use and antibiotics in particular.

How do I know if I have a Candida overgrowth?
The only way to be certain is through testing (such as a stool test) but common signs that a person could be struggling with Candida overgrowth are:

- Frequent bloating
- Constipation or diarrhoea
- Brain fog, difficulty concentrating, mood swings, poor memory, irritability, depression

- Chronic fatigue, or large swings in energy levels
- Strong sugar / carbohydrate cravings
- Fungal infections such as athletes foot and thrush
- Urinary tract infections

What to do in the case of a Candida overgrowth?

If someone does have candida overgrowth then reversing this is very important for clearing up the symptoms and for their long-term health.

Essentially they would need to not only kill the overgrown Candida but also take steps to prevent it coming back again (remember, it grew because conditions weren't as good as they needed to be so fixing the gut is essential).

Therefore, restoring good levels of bacteria, addressing any bad bacteria or parasitic infections, taking steps to remove the factors that reduced good bacteria levels in the first place, and healing the leaky gut, are all important.

The first stage (killing the yeast) will involve starving it through a specialised diet for a short period of time, whilst also using certain anti-fungal supplements to help aid the process. This can be done very quickly and effectively and can make a HUGE difference to how someone feels.

CHAPTER NINE
Phase 2 - Flourish

I fairly recently found out a pretty interesting fact about a friend of mine who I have known for many years. It's something that she had never mentioned before and something which blew my mind. Basically it turns out that her heart is on the wrong side of her body. Did you even know that was possible? I certainly didn't! Everything else is completely in the same, normal place, but her heart is on the right, instead of the left. Apparently it's called Dextrocardia.

It's interesting what you find out about people sometimes isn't it? I always wish I had more interesting facts to tell people about myself (the best I've got is that I once took a wee standing next to Prince William!).

It's a great example of how everyone is completely different, all with our own unique interesting bodies. And because of this, there can never be one perfect protocol or one perfect diet for people with IBD. Everyone will need something slightly different, and personalised towards them. That's a large part of what phase 2 is about as you reintroduce foods to your diet and assess how your body reacts. It can be a really useful way of identifying your own individual sensitivities and, therefore, help to personalise the diet towards you.

It's worth noting that if/when you do identify foods that you are perhaps sensitive to, these aren't necessarily things that will stay with you forever. As you remove them from your diet for a period of time, and as the health of your digestive system improves, and your gut heals, then a lot of your food sensitivities will go away, and your diet can become much more flexible. A lot of my clients are eventually able to eat most things in moderation without getting a reaction. Don't get me wrong, they couldn't eat McDonald's every day and feel great but then again nobody could! But being able to go out for a meal without worrying about how certain foods may affect you is certainly a place that many people can get to.

Reintroducing Foods

After at least 30 days on the Phase 1 diet you can often start reintroducing foods and assess the reaction of the body. However, in the cases where your symptoms have not improved during phase 1, then it likely doesn't make sense to be doing this just yet because clearly there are still underlying problems to be addressed. It may simply be the case that you just need to give it more time (things don't always turn around immediately, especially if you have been ill for a long time). If this does apply to you then don't worry, all your hard work up to now has not been a waste. You should still know that you are doing the right thing. A focus on eating good quality unprocessed foods can only be good for your body. Just because you haven't noticed significant improvements yet, your body will still be much healthier place because of the changes you have made so far, and we are now that much closer to working out what your underlying problems are (remember, it's not just diet that can be a major driver of symptoms).

However, most people will have noticed some level of improvement in Phase 1. For some the improvement will be substantial, for others it will be subtler. If you are happy to continue the diet for a little longer, and don't want to risk adding new foods back in, then that is fine to do so as long as you are eating enough food and aren't losing significant amounts of weight. Make sure you are getting a good variety of foods in though, and a good variety of vegetables especially (provided you can tolerate them). However, if you are finding the diet far too restrictive, or just want a bit more variety in your life, then you will likely relish the opportunity to add some foods back in.

How to reintroduce foods

When reintroducing foods, you should try eating a small amount of the food one day (without making any other substantial changes to your diet), and then wait at least 3 days before testing another food. This will allow you to see if your body has a reaction to the food. Reactions are not always immediate, and don't necessarily result in you rushing to the toilet. If something makes you bloat, gives you reflux, skin problems, or even a change in mood or brain fog then it will be causing you some kind of inflammation and so should be excluded, probably for at least 3 months, before you test reintroducing it again. You should also leave it at least 5 days before testing another food. If you experience an allergic reaction, then you should remove forever. Assuming you don't have any reaction to a food then it is likely going to be ok for you to eat going forward in small quantities, but obviously continue to be aware of any reaction, especially the first few times you eat it.

Personalisation

Following the elimination and reintroduction protocol is a fantastic way of personalising the diet towards you and learning what works best for you and your body. However, if things still aren't great in terms of your health, then it can be worth experimenting with things a little further, dietary wise, to see if they have a benefit. It is all about learning what works for you and while you may have learned what specific foods work for you, further personalisation can occur by playing around with the *types* of foods that you eat and how much of them you eat.

To explain that further, I've listed a few things that you that you may want to try adjusting in your diet to see if it brings added benefit:

- How many starchy carbs you consume each day (some people do better with higher amounts, some with very low amounts).

- How much fat you eat (fats should always be 'good' fats, but some people do better on higher fat diets, some people do better with lower fat)

- How much protein you eat. Some people benefit from a vegetarian type diet, some people do well with a relatively high amount of animal protein in their diet.

- How much fibre you eat (and the types of fibre you eat; insoluble and soluble)

This list, in reality, could go on forever and getting something more detailed and appropriate for you can really be beneficial as it will take out a lot of the guess work for you.

Macronutrients

'Macronutrients' is the collective name for proteins, fats and carbohydrates. These three sections will discuss macronutrients in more detail, and the best sources of these.

Protein

Protein is needed to help your body repair and maintain/build muscle mass. Protein is also very satiating (so helps to better control hunger levels) and is great for helping to control energy throughout the day. The best sources of protein are from meat, fish, and eggs.

Protein Quality

In an ideal world you would get your meat, fish and eggs

from the best possible sources. For example, organic, grass fed meat is the best option when eating meat. If eating salmon, wild salmon is much better than farmed salmon. For eggs, organic, free range eggs are much better than eggs from caged hens. I appreciate that all of these are more expensive options, so only choose them if you feel you can afford it. They aren't essentials to start with. If you find organic meats are too expensive for your budget then it can be worth using local farmers markets or butchers, where the quality can often be a little better than you will get in the major supermarkets. When using these, it can also be worth trying to negotiate deals, particularly if you buy from them regularly or can buy in bulk and use your freezer.

Fats
Fats are extremely important to our health. They are crucial for the production of many of our hormones. They ensure our nervous system functions as it should, and lubricate our cells, allowing for improved nutrient uptake. Therefore, they are crucial for energy and sex drive.

There are good and bad fats, and unfortunately the bad fats have meant that almost all fats have incorrectly been given a bad name. Bad fats, which include things such as vegetable oil and margarine, are often found in processed foods, and used in restaurants for frying, primarily due to the fact they are cheap. They are extremely damaging to your health, can cause heart disease, and increase inflammation in your body.

Obviously digesting fats that you consume is very important as well. One of my old clients Zoe, who is now symptom and medication free, had her gallbladder removed not too long before being diagnosed with ulcerative colitis. One of the first things I put in place with her were specific protocols and supplements to help ensure she was digesting her fats appropriately (which can be problematic because the gall bladder plays a major role in fat digestion). After doing this her symptoms very quickly improved and her energy levels, in particular, were significantly better.

Carbohydrates

Carbs have got a bad name in recent years, partly justified, partly unjustified. You shouldn't avoid carbs (certainly not for long periods of time anyway), you just need to be wise about which carbs you consume, how many you consume, and when you consume them. In today's world many people are prone to consuming large amounts of refined and poor-quality food which has a direct effect on their blood sugar levels. By ensuring the right type and timing of your carbohydrates and ensuring regular servings of protein throughout the day many of the energy related issues will correct themselves.

One thing to be aware of when it comes to energy is that you shouldn't be afraid to eat carbs at night. Doing so will increase your serotonin levels which can help you to relax and get a good quality sleep (which is obviously very important for overcoming fatigue). Those people who are on very low carbs diets often have difficulty sleeping, because they don't have these relaxing carbs in their system.

Eating carbs early in the day (such as with breakfast, which is what many people do) can actually relax you and can lead to a drop in energy. Those foods packed with sugar or high GI carbs will elevate your blood sugar levels, again leading to a mid-morning slump, which can then subsequently mean you attempt to increase your energy levels with more sugar or caffeine. A vicious circle.

CHAPTER TEN
Phase 3 – Fine Tuning Phase

Phase 3 is where subtle changes can dramatically accelerate your progress even further!

By now we have established a good base diet for you, addressed anything underlying in the GI tract, and helped to optimize digestion and absorption, while nourishing your body as much as possible. Therefore, we can now place less focus on the diet and more focus on other areas of your lifestyle that could be compromising your health. In particular, we'll further concentrate on improving the health of your adrenals (which will work wonders for your energy), eliminating any toxins that could be worsening your symptoms, while placing a greater focus on optimising your sleep, stress, mindset and lifestyle to get you firmly on the road to recovery.

Really the principles in this phase should be applied throughout your journey so don't feel like you can forget about them after a little while and just move on to phase 4. The changes here should stay with you for life!

Rest / Sleep
Quality rest and sleep is an often-overlooked component in achieving optimal health, but it can have a huge effect. It is critical for both physical and emotional well-being. Studies have certainly shown that there are links between insufficient sleep and the onset of a flare in Crohn's and Ulcerative Colitis.

If we don't allow our bodies to rest sufficiently, then we cannot expect it to repair and perform at its best. A useful analogy to think about is when people train in the gym to build muscle. The muscle isn't actually built in the gym. In fact, the purpose of the training itself is to stretch, tear and break down the muscle. The muscles can then only repair and grow when they are rested, away from the gym. If all a bodybuilder did was to train and work 24/7, they would never grow any muscles. It's a similar story for you. You need to allow your body to repair. Otherwise it can never begin to perform optimally.

The most important aspect in adequate rest is getting enough sleep. However, it's not everything. You need to consider how much rest you get during the day. Are you always on the go? Do you have a physically demanding job? Do you allow yourself to just have some quality time to sit down and relax?

Sleep, in particular, is crucial for resetting your body. It helps it to heal, regulate the stress response, control blood sugar levels, aids detoxification and improves hormonal and neurotransmitter regulation.

It's also worth remembering the impact that it can have on your hunger and food choices. As you know, consistently eating the right foods for your body is going to be critical for your health and energy. When you don't get enough sleep, your body has too little Leptin and too much Ghrelin. These are 2 hormones within our body. The Leptin is responsible for telling the body that more food is needed, and conversely, a high level tells the body that it doesn't need so much food. Ghrelin is responsible for controlling appetite. Therefore, a drop in Leptin and increase in Ghrelin (which can be caused by lack of sleep), makes you hungrier than you should be, will mess with your metabolism, and ultimately lead to you eating anything and everything that you can get your hands on (which almost certainly won't be healthy!).

Another hormone that is particularly affected by lack of

sleep is testosterone. Ultimately, lower testosterone (caused by poor sleep) will result in lower libido, lower energy and have a detrimental effect on feelings of well-being. When you consider that some of the main symptoms of an IBD sufferer include these elements, you can see that optimising testosterone levels is going to be critical (and therefore, getting enough sleep is critical). And yes, it's an important hormone for men and women.

There's also our friend Cortisol. Lack of sleep can cause an increase in the stress response in our body which ultimately leads to higher cortisol. Cortisol is catabolic and so will inhibit the body's ability to repair. Additionally, it can lead to other stress related issues such as depression, aging and heart problems. Over time, cortisol levels can then drop, which will affect energy, and can cause inflammation problems. What's more, changes in our cortisol levels can affect our blood sugar levels - and as you may remember, effective blood sugar management is one of our pillars of health that we are working on. Therefore, keeping cortisol in balance is important.

Following on from the above, if we are not effectively controlling our blood sugar levels then this can affect our cortisol levels, and an increase in cortisol when we are asleep can mean we wake up.

Many people disrupt their sleep to get up in the night to go to the toilet. However, going to the toilet quite often isn't the reason that they wake up, but they think they might as well go because they are awake. Normally the waking is due to another problem (a stress response or blood sugar fluctuation) in the body and addressing whatever it is that is stressing it will be important.

The amount of sleep that each person needs is very specific to that person (though I believe you should be aiming for 7-8 hours as a very general rule).

There are obviously many tips and tricks to help optimise your sleep. I have helped some of my clients who don't remember sleeping through the night in years get a completely restful night's sleep in a matter of days with some simple changes.

Environment (Stress)

Stress is described in Merriam Webster's medical dictionary as "a physical, chemical or emotional factor that causes bodily or mental tension and may be a factor in disease causation; a state of bodily or mental tension resulting from factors that tend to alter an existent equilibrium".

Stress can be either 'distress' or 'eustress', which are both very different. Eustress is a positive effect on the body – something that you would experience perhaps when you are doing something exhilarating. Distress is a negative type of stress and can be described as any influence, internal or external, that causes or leads to malfunction.

The impact of (di)stress on our health should never be underestimated. Almost all the IBD sufferers I have known and worked with over the years have all seen an increase in their symptoms when they are going through a period of stress. What's more, for most them, if they have ever been able to identify a 'trigger' that they felt initially brought on their IBD when they were first diagnosed, then it was a stressful event or period in their life - exams, moving to a new house, divorce, the death of a loved one. Whatever it is, it has caused them some stress and that has certainly contributed towards the onset of their illness. Someone could have the best diet in the world, yet if they were chronically stressed then their health would suffer.

A little stress in our lives isn't necessarily a bad thing. Our bodies are designed to cope with stressful events. Our Paleolithic ancestors, for example, would have been stressed if they were being chased by a tiger. That would have raised their cortisol and prepared their bodies for 'fight or flight'. But once that stressful event was over, their bodies would have returned to a normal state of ease. How times have changed though. Now we worry about meetings, deadlines, presentations, getting the kids to school, not enough time for sleep or relaxation, physical stress from over-training, worrying what someone thinks of us, trying to reply to all our emails, check our FB status, how many followers we have, and so on. Many people live in a constant state of stress, i.e. chronic stress. Our bodies just aren't designed for this.

This constant bombardment of stressors places a large demand on our adrenal glands, and eventually it adversely impacts their function which has a knock-on effect to our overall health. The adrenal glands affect so much and without optimal function of the adrenals we cannot expect to function optimally as a whole. Interferences and imbalances in one area of the body will always have ripple effect on to other areas in the body.

Another important area impacted by chronically high stress levels is our digestion. This is for several reasons, one major one being that, because we are in a constant state of 'fight or flight', our bodies are moving blood to the areas where it will be most needed for a fight or flight response. Digesting food optimally is not essential at the moment in time you are being chased by a tiger. So, if our body constantly thinks it's in a state of stress (such as being chased by a tiger), then it will fail to digest its food properly. The impact that this could have on your IBD, your bowel movements, and your nutrient absorption is huge and will certainly be a contributor towards fatigue.

Whilst this obviously isn't directly related to IBD as such, one final interesting point on stress is that studies into pregnancies have shown that conceptions are particularly high during holiday periods. Yes, a time when we relax, unwind and for once in our lives forget about the daily worries. Basically, in a constant state of stress, we even find it difficult to reproduce! And then when we do manage to get pregnant, a period of stress through the pregnancy has been shown to be a major factor in miscarriage and impaired foetal development. If stress can have this impact on our ability to reproduce, then there can be no doubt whatsoever that it is severely impacting our overall health and wellbeing.

For the body composition concerned amongst you, it's also worth mentioning that high stress levels are strongly correlated with excess fat around the abdominal area. So, if you have some love handles you want to lose, there's even more incentive for you to keep stress under control!

Stressors to the body can be 'internal' and 'external'. Internal stressors, such as food sensitivities, poor detoxification, poor digestion, hidden infections, etc are primarily addressed, identified and resolved using the appropriate diet, lifestyle supplementation and testing (all discussed in other areas of this book).   External stressors are things such as arguments with people, rushing to meet deadlines, relationship troubles, financial stress, etc. It is your response to these events, as well as minimising the number of these events that you are exposed to, that will determine the level of external stress in your life.

Environment (Toxins)
Did you know that by the time you leave the house in the

morning, you may have already been exposed to around 15 toxins? That's before you even step out of the door into the car fumes outside!

Toxins are all around us, from the water we drink, the products we use, the medications that we take, even from some clothing that we wear. And they can seriously impact our health. There is rightly a lot of focus on the food we put into our body, but these toxins are all still entering our body, both through our mouth as well as being absorbed through the skin.

Minimising toxin exposure could be a whole book in itself but to summarise, carefully considering the products that you put on to your skin, that you eat out of, that you drink out of, that you clean your house with and wash your clothes with are all important and can help put a much lower strain on the detoxification required in your body.

Activity / Exercise

As you will no doubt be aware, the right activity / exercise is important for everyone's health.

The benefits of exercise are wide ranging; it helps to improve blood flow, aids cardiovascular fitness and overall health, while improving feelings of wellbeing through the release of endorphins. Additionally, it can help to aid detoxification as your body will release toxins when you sweat. There can also (depending on your chosen sport/exercise) be a valuable (often *under-valued*) social side to exercise. Regular social interaction and support can be critical for everyone and is especially needed when suffering with something such as IBD (even though at times it can tempting to "just want to be alone for a while").

However, to truly experience the benefits of exercise there

are a few things you should be careful of:

1) you mustn't do too much exercise (especially when you suffer with IBD)
2) you do the right type of exercise for your body and your goals

Too Much Exercise

Too much exercise, if suffering with your health, can lead to 'over-training' which can be a physical stressor on the body (physical and mental stress is very important to keep under control when living with IBD). With too much exercise, you put your body under too much strain. Your body needs to be allowed to rest and recover and if it has to do too much in the way of physical activity, then it won't be able to do that sufficiently.

Over-training has been shown to lead to feelings of depression and chronic fatigue by influencing blood levels of glutamine, dopamine and 5-HTP, and can affect hormone production.

Over-training can also adversely affect the immune system and has even been linked with the development of autoimmune conditions such as IBD. A good way to judge if you are doing too much can be to assess how you feel after the exercise. If you feel good, then what you are doing is probably OK. If you feel shattered, drained, and unable to do much else for the rest of the day, then you have done too much, and you should drastically reduce how much you are doing. Other signs of over-training include feeling run down, frequent colds, losing muscle mass, and gaining fat despite eating well.

You should also consider how active you are in day to day life, away from formal 'exercise'. For example, if you have a demanding physical job, then you will likely have even less energy available for additional exercise. It might be that the job alone is too much and if it leaves you shattered at the end of the day, then seeking alternative employment or roles may be appropriate for your long-term health.

The Wrong Kind of Exercise

Different types of exercise can have different effects on the body. Certain types of exercise will be more likely than others to take the body to a place of physical exhaustion which can do much more harm than good. If someone goes for a leisurely walk, then this will obviously not place anywhere near as much stress on the body as running a marathon would, for example.

Perhaps less obvious is that something such as a 100m sprint has a different effect on the body as perhaps a 5-mile jog. Even though the 100m sprint may leave you feeling even more out of breath than the 5-mile jog, you are actually placing the body under a lower level of chronic stress and, in general (not always), our bodies are better able to cope with quick high intensity bouts of sprinting than they are with lower intensity, long periods of exercise.

That's not to say you should never jog again – I just want to make the point that if you suffer with IBD you should be wary, in particular, of doing too much low intensity steady state periods of exercise. However, as per above, a good way to judge what's right for you is how the exercise leaves you feeling afterward. Getting in tune with your body is really important here. One way to do that is through monitoring heart rate variability (discussed more below)

So, What Should I Do?

This will depend on what stage you feel you are at with your IBD. If you are flaring, or feeling pretty run down, then I would suggest you limit your exercise to leisurely walks each day (perhaps 20-30 mins long, out in the country if possible, and gradually increase intensity/distance as and when you start to feel better). Perhaps you could also do some yoga or pilates type exercises which can be great for the body <u>and</u> mind.

The decision on what you do is obviously your call and I would suggest listening to your body and making a judgment about where you are currently with your IBD and your symptoms.

Finally, getting adequate rest and sleep after any kind of physical activity is crucial.

I have worked with many clients who have completed triathlons, marathons, and 100-mile bike rides. But it wasn't always the case that they were able to do these things. They suffered badly too with fatigue at one point and had to dramatically reduce how much exercise they did (which wasn't always easy for them because it's something they loved). But very quickly we were able to turn things around, and their activity levels were able to increase, enabling them start living the life they love again.

<u>Magnesium</u>

There are numerous supplements that may be beneficial to introduce at this stage, but it really would be decided on a case by case basis. However, one that is worthy of consideration is Magnesium. Magnesium is one of the most abundant minerals in the body and is critical for many functions. We can obtain magnesium from our food but due to modern farming methods, the amount we can obtain is getting lower meaning that many people are becoming deficient. It can be a worthwhile supplement to introduce at this phase as it can aid energy production, maintain blood pressure, aid sleep, improve recovery, and support the adrenals.

Magnesium can also be especially worthwhile using if you ever find you are constipated, but for this reason it may not be appropriate to use certain types of magnesium if you are still having urgent or frequent bowel movements.

CHAPTER TWELVE
Phase 4 - Rebuilding

In this phase we will be rebuilding and repairing the health of your gut. Your gut is designed to help absorb nutrients from the foods we eat, whilst acting as a barrier against excessive absorption of things such as bacteria and toxins. However, because of previous problems, it has likely become damaged over the years.

The work done in the previous phases will have removed a lot of the inflammatory foods and pathogens that are damaging the gut but the damage will have been done and so we need to start to repair things. To do this we'll use specific foods and additional supplements (for a short period) to help do this.

As you work to heal your gut you will likely notice a dramatic improvement in symptoms, your energy levels will be higher than they have been in ages, and many of your food sensitivities start to go away (eventually allowing for increased flexibility within the diet).

Leaky Gut

"Leaky gut" or "intestinal permeability" is very heavily linked with autoimmune conditions such as Crohn's or Ulcerative Colitis. Some people would suggest that to have an autoimmune condition you MUST have a leaky gut, but it now appears that's not necessarily the case (though it's pretty damn likely). The small intestine helps to absorb nutrients from the foods we eat, as well as acting as a barrier against excessive absorption of things such as bacteria and toxins.

When a gut is 'leaky', undigested food particles and things such as parasites, bacteria, fungi and toxic wastes (that would normally be eliminated), are allowed to pass through the intestinal barrier into the blood stream. These will then be recognised by the body as an invader and the immune system will attack it. The immune system response can result in a large number of symptoms including joint pain, frequent toilet visits, poor energy, and depression.

Why does a gut become leaky?
A leaky gut will normally occur due to inflammation. It can be caused by a huge number of factors including:

- medication
- alcohol
- chronic stress (physical or mental)
- non-steroidal anti-inflammatory drugs
- infections
- food intolerances/allergies.

The inflammation caused by these factors puts pressure on the gut wall and makes it permeable (i.e. "leaky"). The steps that we take, especially in the early stages of the 5 Phase Thrive, are primarily aimed at removing these potential causes. Once that is done we can then place a greater focus on healing the gut.

How do I know if my gut is leaky?
As mentioned previously, it is fairly certain (though not 100%) that if you have IBD and aren't in complete, drug free remission, then your gut is very likely 'leaky'. However, there are tests that allow you to be certain. I discuss those more in Phase 5.

What are the effects of a leaky gut?
The immune system response can affect various tissues in the body and stimulate an inflammatory reaction in that area, resulting in a large number of symptoms. If that inflammatory

reaction occurs within the gut lining, the result may be (depending on numerous other factors, including genetics) Crohn's or Ulcerative Colitis.

Perhaps you suffer badly with joint pain or rheumatoid arthritis (which is certainly very common in those who suffer with IBD)? Well this can mean that the leaky gut has ultimately also led to an inflammatory reaction in your joints. In reality the reaction can take in numerous areas of the body and, therefore, result in a range of symptoms (this is one reason why we often say that all disease starts in the gut). Even depression (again, a common problem for those with IBD) has its roots in the gut.

Additionally, a leaky gut can cause numerous other problems:

- It will vastly increase the number of foods to which you are sensitive or intolerant

- It will put a lot of burden on the liver, as it tries to detoxify the antigens that are making their way into the blood stream.

- Studies have suggested the when a pregnant woman has a leaky gut, then the healthy development of her offspring could be compromised.

How do I heal my leaky gut?
As already mentioned, the first step is to make sure you have removed anything that could be causing the gut to be "leaky" in the first place (so problem foods, toxins, parasites, bad bacteria, stress must all be addressed, which is why the first 3 phases of the 5 Phase Thrive are critical to complete before getting to this phase). Without doing that it would be completely pointless trying to repair the gut while you are still damaging it.

It's worth remembering that most of your food sensitivities and intolerances exist for a reason and, quite often, that reason is a leaky gut. People who do repair their leaky gut find that not only will a huge amount (if not all) of their symptoms go away, but so will many of their food sensitivities. Removing foods without working to help the body to heal makes long term health very difficult. It would likely mean you are forever fighting a losing battle, with your diet becoming consistently more restrictive. Bone broth, organ meat and certain supplements (including Saccharomyces Boulardii, Glutamine, and Collagen) can help to you to get there (though aren't necessarily suitable for everyone).

CHAPTER THIRTEEN
Phase 5 – Thrive for Life

By now you will likely be thriving, feeling like a new person, with so much more energy, and very little sign of symptoms. The plans we will put in place in this phase will help to build on that and keep you fit and healthy forever!

In particular, we will help to improve the level of good bacteria within your gut which can have significant impact on your health and re-educate your immune system to function as it should.

I'll also discuss some testing to help identify if you could be on course for a relapse/flare (sorry "Blip") and if so what to do about it.

Bacteria
The right blend of bacteria in your gut is critical for overall health and energy levels. You may have heard about how your gut can contain both good and bad bacteria. This is very true, and, in fact, you have more bacteria within your body than cells (it's in the trillions)

There are many factors, especially in this day and age, that can cause an imbalance in your gut bacteria.

What affects our bacteria levels?
Antibiotics are certainly a huge factor because they essentially kill off the bacteria within your gut, whether that be good or bad. Destroying your good bacteria is certainly NOT something you want to be doing at any time, especially if you suffer with IBD. Our good bacteria can virtually be completed eliminated by a single course of antibiotics and even

years later our gut bacteria can still be disrupted after the antibiotic use. This is why I'm hesitant to use antibiotics unless it's really necessary (which it can sometimes be), and almost always recommend that someone supplements for a short period of time with a quality probiotic (good bacteria) and saccharomyces boulardii during and after using antibiotics. It is my strong belief that one major cause of the massively high chronic disease rates across the western world (and the ever-increasing rates of IBD) are the overuse of antibiotics, especially from a very early age.

Aside from antibiotics, other drivers of imbalanced gut flora include:

- Drugs / Medication
- Poor diet
- Consuming foods you are intolerant or sensitive towards
- Contraception
- Stress
- Toxin exposure
- If you were breast fed
- If you were born naturally or via C section.
- Our levels of cleanliness (see below)

Cleanliness
Research has shown that contact with farm animals when you were growing up has been linked with up to a 50% reduced risk of getting IBD. Clearly, something about being on the farm, or around farm animals, somehow strengthens the immune system. But what?

One of the studies only showed a benefit to those who were born after 1952. Before then, there appears to be no difference whether you grew up on a farm or in the city. So, what's so magical about that date? Well nothing about the year in particular but it's a sign of gradually changing times as the differences between the "microbial environment" of cities and the countryside have increased over the last century. People who live in more urban areas are being exposed to far fewer bacteria (which is why little differences were noted many years ago, but the effects are becoming more prominent now).

This line of thinking is related to something known as "the Hygiene Hypothesis" which shows that exposure to germs / dirt / bacteria from a young age can actually HELP to reduce the chance of illness in later life. It is thought that it does this by strengthening the immune system and improving the health of our microbiome, in particular the mix of good and bad bacteria in our guts. Basically, it would seem that being too obsessed with cleanliness, especially in our early years, can actually be a bad thing.

Probiotic Foods

Certain foods are high in levels of good bacteria and incorporating some of these into your diet can be extremely beneficial. A few of these foods are details below:

Sauerkraut

Sauerkraut (which is basically a fermented white cabbage) can be a fantastically tasty (and healthy) addition to your meals. As long as you buy the right one (go for 'raw and unpasteurised') eating sauerkraut will fill your gut with beneficial bacteria which is vital to your overall health and wellbeing (similar to taking a probiotic supplement). Finding the right kind isn't as easy as it should be (most supermarkets won't sell it). You can often get it in a Polish shop if you have one near you or buy some online. Alternatively, you may decide to make your own.

Kefir

Kefir is a fermented milk product that contains numerous

beneficial bacteria. Even if someone has problems consuming dairy they are normally (not always) ok with Kefir because it has been fermented. Kefir is a good source of calcium, magnesium, phosphorus and B vitamins. You can also make your own kefir, including water kefir if you do not consume dairy.

Intestinal Permeability (Leaky Gut) Testing

A leaky gut test isn't necessarily something that I would use straight away with someone (because unless you are in drug free remission it is almost certain you do have a leaky gut so we don't need to test for it). However, once someone is in drug free (or minimal medication) remission then an annual or bi-annual test can be worthwhile as it can provide a warning sign of if your health is slowly worsening (it's been shown that a gut may be 'leaky' up to a year prior to the onset of symptoms, and so we can help to prevent flares before they happen). If you find that you do have a leaky gut, then you can put in place protocols to address things before your symptoms show themselves.

One good test has you drink a sugary solution that contains molecules called Lactulose and Mannitol. The test measures the ability of these sugar molecules to pass through the intestinal lining. A few hours after drinking you provide a urine sample which is sent to the lab who can test for the levels of lactulose and mannitol found in your urine and gain a better understand not just of how "leaky" your gut is but also how well it can absorb smaller molecules that should be able to pass through (thus indicating how well you are able to absorb nutrients from the foods you eat).

Lactulose is the larger of the molecules. If lactulose is elevated (out of range) in the urine it indicates that there is increased permeability between the cells ("paracellular") which we don't want.

Mannitol is the smaller of the molecules. Mannitol recovery is looking at the speed at which small molecules move through the cells (in the way that nutrients from food would). The levels of this help us to understand the *condition* of the cells of the gut. A low Mannitol reading can mean that things aren't being correctly absorbed which longer term could lead to numerous problems, including fatigue (a very common problem for IBD sufferers). This type of result can indicate some damage to the lining of the gut which means that it isn't absorbing these molecules (or nutrients) as well as it perhaps should. There are tiny little villi on the lining of the gut responsible for this absorption and when damaged are like a shaggy carpet where bits can get worn away.

As I said this can be a good test to regularly do once you are symptom and medication free (or close to it). Another test that can be a sign that your health is worsening is a stool test which would show inflammatory markers.

CHAPTER FOURTEEN
Frequently Asked Questions

That brings us to the end of the 5 Phase Thrive but I'm sure you may have some questions, many of which I have hopefully addressed below…

Why am I getting reflux / heart burn?

Something that's not always appreciated is that a common cause of reflux actually isn't high stomach acid, as most people believe, but rather stomach acid being too low. Not always, but quite often. However, unfortunately many millions of people each year are being put on acid suppressing drugs without their doctors performing simple tests to understand if they are *really* needed. I've seen just how overused these drugs are with some of my private clients where at least 2 of them had previously been put on acid suppressing drugs "just in case they got reflux" (which is a known side effect of other medications they are on). How crazy is that!?

A large amount of the confusion comes about because these drugs do often provide short term relief for someone who is suffering with reflux. This is because it *is* stomach acid finding its way in to the oesophagus that brings on the symptoms of acid reflux, and so suppressing that stomach acid helps to relieve the symptoms (temporarily). But then the question comes "why was the stomach acid getting into the oesophagus in the first place?". When we look at the most common answer to this question it appears that these drugs are generally making things much worse, in the long term, because it's thought that low stomach acid is actually the cause of the issues.

How can low stomach acid be the real cause?

Low stomach acid causes many problems that ultimately put pressure on the lower oesophageal sphincter (LES). The LES is meant to act as a barrier between the oesophagus and the stomach, essentially designed help keep the stomach acid out. But because of all the pressure that is built up in the stomach (ultimately caused by the low stomach acid meaning that food is not being appropriately digested) the LES malfunctions and opens, thus allowing acid into the oesophagus.

What are the symptoms?

Signs that your stomach acid may be too low include acid reflux, bloating, gas, burping, and heartburn. Feeling particularly uncomfortable or nauseous after a meal (when eating meat in particular) can certainly be a good indicator.

Why is it important to address?

Proper stomach acid levels are critical for our digestive processes, as well as being important for our immune system. Low stomach acid (hypochlorhydria) is a commonly overlooked problem linked with numerous illnesses and diseases including autoimmune conditions (such as IBD), SIBO, asthma and stomach cancer, and can very much be a cause of fatigue.

Stomach acid is needed to help break down our foods (proteins in particular), which is why if you feel uncomfortable, bloated, gassy etc. after eating then this can indicate low levels (and one reason that I believe many people feel that they can't eat red meat – not because there is a problem with the meat itself but more because they don't have enough acid to break it down sufficiently). Just like if you don't chew your food properly you can get digestive problems, if you don't have sufficient stomach acid levels you can again experience problems.

Optimal stomach acid is extremely important for nutrient absorption (iron, B12, folate, zinc and calcium especially) and could be one reason that many IBD sufferers are deficient in iron and B12 in particular (and, therefore, fatigue). Acid in the stomach is also used not just for breaking down food but for helping to quickly kill bacteria and other bugs/infections that enter the body (so is an important part of our immune system).

Testing

There are a few ways to test your stomach acid levels. The simplest one to do from home is using a Betaine HCL supplement. If doing this you should do under the care of someone who knows what they are doing, but essentially you take some Betaine HCL (always a product with Pepsin), eat a meal containing a good amount of protein/meat, and during the meal take one Betaine HCL tablet. Finish your meal and pay attention to how you feel. If you don't notice anything then it could mean that your stomach acid levels are too low. If you notice a burning sensation in your stomach, then this can be a good sign that your stomach acid levels are appropriate. It's not a completely fool proof test but it can be a good indicator.

So, what can be done?

Firstly, supplementation is always an option to help bring your stomach acid levels back to where they need to be. Again, I don't advise mindlessly supplementing, you should always consult a professional when doing this. Supplementation should only be a short-term strategy though – it shouldn't be something you look to rely on forever, as it doesn't really address the cause of the low stomach acid in the first place. Stress, medication, diets high in sugar, gluten, wheat, alcohol and processed foods, antibiotic use, infections (H-Pylori in particular), and bacterial overgrowth are all thought to be potential causes and addressing them is critical for long term health.

Like I said, low stomach acid isn't the only cause of reflux, but it is certainly one that seems to be especially common, and when you understand that you see just how insane it is that millions of people each year are being given medication that is very likely to be making things worse in the long term.

Should I be avoiding all animal fats?

It is not uncommon for certain people to suggest that you should leave all animal fats out of your diet for optimal health. However, this is not true.

Firstly, you need to be very careful of allowing your overall fat intake to go too low, especially if you plan on having a smidgen of sex drive and energy each day. As already mentioned, fat intake is critical for overcoming fatigue.

Obviously not all good fats are directly from meat, and some fatty meats *are* best avoided, but that certainly doesn't mean that *all* of them should be cut out. When considering which meats are ok and which aren't, one thing to consider is what did the animal eat when it was alive? Some animals will eat lots of toxins in their lifetime (mainly found in the poor food they get fed). When this happens, those toxins are stored in the animal's fat cells, and by the time we come to eat that animal those toxins are still stored in the fat in the meat. As an example, pigs are generally fed pretty much anything and everything when they are alive, which ultimately leads to the meat (especially bacon) being of lower quality, with high levels of toxins in the fat. Therefore, when eating bacon, it's well worth trimming off the fat. But if you compare that to say an organic grass-fed steak, then it's a significantly different situation and almost certainly the fats within it will be fine and perfectly healthy for you.

Therefore, rather than believing you need to cut out all fatty meats, instead pay more attention to the quality of the meat you are eating. Remember you are not what you eat, but what you eat has eaten.

I've heard that I need to avoid fibre. Is this true?

Here's a quote from Wikipedia regarding the low residue (low fibre) diet…

"New evidence tends to run counter to the well-established myth that a low residue diet is beneficial. A Mayo Clinic review from 2011 finds no evidence for the superiority of low residue diets in treating diverticular disease and in fact tends to show that a high-fibre diet can prevent diverticular disease. A systematic review published in 2012 found no high-quality studies but found that some studies and guidelines favour a high-fibre diet for the treatment of symptomatic disease."

Yet despite these studies, 1000's of IBD patients every year are told it is beneficial. Low residue normally means 2 things happen:

1. Someone cuts ALL fruit and vegetables out of their diet, because of this overwhelming fear of all fibre.

2. Someone eats lots and lots of white bread because it's one of the few things allowed (despite the fact that so many people are sensitive or intolerant to gluten and wheat).

If you are on a "low residue diet", then I would urge you to look elsewhere as it's rarely the long-term solution to your health problems. Now don't get me wrong, the amount of fibre that someone eats can be a problem sometimes in specific cases. However, at the same time fibre is also very important for the healthy functioning of the gut. It can help to regulate the consistency of the stools and make the passing of them much easier. It also has a large influence on the growth of friendly bacteria in the gut and helps to control blood sugar levels.

Dietary fibre is the indigestible portion of food derived from plants and waste of animals that eat dietary fibre. It remains intact through the gastrointestinal tract, meaning it has a cleansing function within the body. Fibre is essential for ensuring gastrointestinal health and plays a huge role in the prevention of disease. It helps to change the nature of the contents of the GI tract and how other nutrients and chemicals are absorbed. There are two different types of fibre – soluble and insoluble. This basically refers to whether or not they dissolve in water (soluble being the one that does). The two types play different roles, but both are important.

Soluble fibre is found in things such as oats, legumes, and some nuts (especially almonds), fruit (such as berries) and vegetables (including broccoli). They form a gel like consistency within the gut and tend to slow the movement of food in the system. It, therefore, can help to improve blood sugar regulation, satiety and would ideally be consumed at times when rapid digestion of foods is not required. The downside is that overconsumption can lead to constipation.

Insoluble fibre is different. Found in foods such as leafy greens, sweet potato, whole grains, certain fruits (such as avocado), and many nuts and seeds, it tends to accelerate the digestive process and, therefore, helps to keep you regular. It adds bulk to stool and allows them to pass through the gut more easily, although certain studies have demonstrated excess insoluble fibre may be harmful to the gut by being a potential irritant to an already inflamed gut lining, fuelling the growth of opportunistic bacteria, and preventing nutrients from being absorbed.

Fibre, and different types of fibre, will have differing effects on different people. In particular, people who suffer with

Crohn's can sometimes develop strictures and in these cases insoluble fibre may need to be reduced (when inflammation is elevated). It can also sometimes be sensible to reduce the amount of insoluble fibre you eat when you are in a flare. However, removing or reducing fibre completely should rarely be done for the long term because it is so important for your overall health. The digestion of soluble fibre produces short chain fatty acids, one of which is butyrate. Butyrate is the primary fuel source for the cells of the intestine, and so is extremely important and can be very effective for sufferers of IBD. It has been shown to be beneficial in reducing inflammation and reducing the chances of cancer in the GI tract. With a very low fibre diet, it is highly likely that your short chain fatty acid, and butyrate, levels would be very low, which is obviously not good for long term health. Therefore, I do not recommend a low residue diet, certainly not for the long term.

CHAPTER FIFTEEN
Resources

Book Bonuses
For access to some free resources that perfectly accompany this book, including a one page cheat sheet, more useful tips on the diet and some very powerful mindset and stress reducing based exercises then just click head here
http://iamgregwilliams.com/book-bonuses-join/

Website
My site, at which I blog on a regular basis, and which includes more information about myself, my work, and my range of products and services is http://iamgregwilliams.com/

Success Stories
For a selection of success stories of IBD sufferers who have completely turned their health around then visit
http://iamgregwilliams.com/success-stories/

Supplements
For a range of very high quality, effective, pure supplements, then head to https://autoimmuneinstitute.com/

CHAPTER SIXTEEN
Conclusion and Success Stories

I hope you have found the enclosed informative and useful and has helped to give you hope that there may be a better way and that you haven't been sentenced to a lifetime of suffering simply because you have been diagnosed with Crohn's or Ulcerative Colitis. I wish you all the best in your journey to better health and a better life. The combination of my 5 Phase Thrive and DREAMT principles can, if followed, completely transform your health and energy levels when living with Crohn's or Ulcerative Colitis.

I love to hear your success stories and would love to be kept up to date with how this book has helped you achieve your health goals!

If you haven't yet done so already, please do remember to head over to this webpage where you can claim some free resources that will accompany the book.

http://www.iamgregwilliams.com/book-bonuses-join/

In good health,

Greg Williams
www.IamGregWilliams.com

p.s. if you have enjoyed this book I'd really appreciate you leaving a 5 star review on Amazon, as it really helps to spread the word about the book and gives other IBD sufferers the opportunity to turn their health around. Thank you so much!

p.p.s. I'd like to leave you with a few more success stories to help give you inspiration that it is possible to turn things around when you take the approach I have shared in this book…

"I was diagnosed with Crohn's in October 2007, following a year of cramps, diarrhoea & sickness. I suffered badly at least once a year from that moment onwards, each year resulted in hospitalisation, with the exception of a short period of remission whilst I was pregnant in 2011.

Over that time I was given lots of drugs including Prednisolone, Azathioprine and Infliximab. However, they weren't making me feel any better and I hated putting them in my body. I was eating a very good diet, full of unprocessed foods but it still wasn't helping.

I reached out to Greg for help and it has completely changed my life. My inflammation levels have reduced significantly and I have been able to eliminate my medication which was a major goal of mine. What's more I feel absolutely fantastic!

Honestly, if you suffer with IBD then I would highly recommend getting in touch with Greg – I'm so glad that I did as I feel amazing and it's transformed my health." - **Kayleigh Vermont**

"I was diagnosed with Crohn's about 18yrs ago, though my symptoms started about a year or two before that.

In particular, I suffered with bloating, pain in the stomach, and especially sharp pains on the right side, and also nausea. I was going to the toilet far too often, but my biggest frustration was the lack of energy. I wasn't able to exercise as much as I would like and wasn't able to do as much as I wanted with my children because I felt so shattered.

I was heading towards 40 and decided there was no better time to start turning things around, which is why I got in touch with Greg.

I'm so glad I did. Over the past 6 months I've worked with him and Colin (one of his coaches) and feel so so so much better. My bowel movements are now back under control, and I have so much more energy now to do the things I love including exercise and spending more time with my family.

What's more I enjoy everything about my diet and lifestyle. I had been a bit hesitant about getting in touch with Greg as I was concerned I'd be put on a boring, restrictive diet, but I genuinely do love what I eat and know I will be able to do this for the rest of my life.

Honestly, if you suffer with Crohns or Ulcerative Colitis and want to get your life back, then get in touch with Greg. Im so glad that I did, it will make a massive difference to how you feel." - **Tim Peters**

"When I first approached Greg in April 2015 I was struggling badly with fatigue and stomach pains which led to poor concentration, night sweats and low energy levels. It had pretty much been like that since I was diagnosed with Crohn's 2 years before.

Being a very sporty person, life was frustrating not being able to perform to the best of my abilities or able to summon the energy when I wanted to be playing sport.

I was hesitant at first to get in touch with Greg because there is a lot of bad advice online but I'm so glad that I did. Doing so has completely changed my health.

My symptoms have reduced dramatically, I've reduced my medication, and feel so much more energetic.

Where my energy levels peaked and troughed, they now remain at a constant higher level. I'm now eager to play sports again without the restraints that Crohn's seemed to have imposed on me and recently completed a 100 mile bike ride. I play hockey regularly and also enjoy endurance outdoor swimming!

I enjoy the food I eat and while changes were obviously needed, it was nowhere near as hard as I thought it would be.

Another side effect I discovered about my new diet is how I no longer look at food and do not want to eat it. I have a much greater appetite and love eating again.

*All I can say to anyone thinking of getting in touch with Greg is to just do it – it can help you to very quickly feel so much better and let you live your life again without many of the symptoms of a debilitating disease." - **Alistair Pettefer***

"When I got diagnosed with Crohn's disease after a couple of years of badgering the GP to send me for some tests I was told I only had a 'mild' form of Crohn's.

This meant that whilst I still got stomach pains, bloating, constipation and fatigue, I didn't have it as bad as others. This is the reason why despite being told by a few different Doctors and Consultants that I should go on medication I didn't. I weighed it up and decided that I could cope with the pains and tiredness as they weren't as bad as the potential side effects of medication.

Fast forward a few months of constant pain and tiredness and the side effects of medication started to look more appealing than the constant daily battle I was having.

Aside from the physical symptoms I found that I was always feeling like I was complaining, complaining I was tired, complaining I was bloated, complaining that I had to go to work or go out when in fact all I wanted to do was nothing but lie on the sofa.

This obviously also had a massive impact on my husband Neil, who wanted 'the old Lynzi back' (probably the worst thing that could be said to someone suffering like this- not that he was to know).

The day I decided something had to change was a day where I'd been battling the pain most of the day and had a gym class in the evening. Driving to the gym I realised I was so tired and in so much pain that I couldn't even contemplate getting changed for the class, never mind the hour of exercise that followed it and sobbed all the way home (not because of missing the class but because I knew I couldn't carry on fighting this battle every day).

The next day I started some googling and found Greg through his website and twitter. I did some research and decided to give him a call. I knew I needed to do something that wasn't medication related but didn't know what it was.

Within weeks of working with him I felt so much better. Yes it was hard cutting out certain foods and planning every meal but it got so much easier.

Greg is really easy to talk to and supportive and gave me all the tools I needed to make myself feel better for the long term rather than quick fixes.

I recently went out for a drink with my best friend on a Friday night after a long week at work and still had bags of energy, I knew I'd done the right thing working with Greg when she told me that it was great to see how energetic I was and how a few months before I would have been too tired to go out.

I often work quite long days and its brilliant that I'm not shattered by 2pm and counting the minutes until I can be reunited with my sofa. Things like this can seem like a massive investment but it's definitely the best investment I've ever made! I would encourage everyone to contact Greg and get started on a plan like this as I genuinely don't think you would regret it." - **Lynzi Agar**

"I was diagnosed with severe Ulcerative Colitis in 2005. I was given massive amounts of anti inflammatory tablets, at first they worked, I was back to normal, but predictably after a while my symptoms worsened. I tried everything. I did lead a stressful life and when my husband had a stroke it became unbearable, still I carried on not wanting to let him down or to be at the mercy of a care home, after he died, I went down with everything, chest infections, aching, extreme tiredness and lots of other nasty symptoms from head to foot.

In July of 2016, feeling so ill and ready to roll over and join my man, after all at 72yrs what was there to live for , flare after flare turned into one long illness. I just could not get well, I was depressed and in so much pain, couldn't eat much without feeling worse.

I was scrolling Facebook and found Greg, he was the only person who's message gave hope, instead of the usual fire fighting of all other disciplines. When I contacted him I did ask him if he was a charlatan. That couldn't have been further from the truth.

The process was all encompassing at first, so much to learn, but so much fun. I found a reason to live again and felt so well, within a few short weeks I truly felt better and looked better than I have done for years. My friends said they had got the old Val back, what a compliment.

I achieved so much from the program, new insight to foods that harm and those that heal. How to look after myself in ways I had not felt like doing even if I knew about them. Feeling well after 12 yrs of pain and illness, being able to come off the medication which I know damage kidneys and liver. I look so good now as I've lost all the blubber that came with my health being out of control. I can't do much about the wrinkles but I can now get into clothes I've not been able to wear for years , I look slim, smart and feel so confident. I am symptom free !!!

My advice to anyone with Crohns or Ulcerative Colitis, don't waste time and money anywhere else. You are guided and supported ever step of the course, with Greg you never feel alone, you are part of a family. You can ask any questions they are always addressed with understanding and care. I have just finished the course and feel wonderful thanks to you Greg." - **Valerie Boller**

"I began working with Greg Williams in December 2015. I am 42 years old and had been struggling with UC for 6-7 years. At that point in time my ulcerative colitis was as bad as it had ever been. It was highly debilitating. I would have 10-12 BMs a day, could never sleep more than 2-3 hours a night (if you could even call it sleep), and was always fatigued. I would have to wait for a "window of time" between BMs just to try to drive to work each morning!

Over the years I had gone through many periods on Prednisone and had also taken Lialda and 6MP for a couple years. In early 2015, after many failures on the previously mentioned meds, I was put on Humira. While on Humira, not only did my symptoms persist, or even worsen, but I was losing weight rapidly and would feel nauseous for at least 4-5 days after each injection. I would decline pretty much all social interaction with friends and family because I was too weak, and didn't know when a flare would occur.

After following Greg on Twitter for a few months, I decided to reach out to him. In looking at his posts, he obviously knew what I was going through, so even though he was in England and I was in the US, I took the chance. I mean at this point, what was there to lose? In my first consultation, Greg and I discussed how I was feeling, what meds I was on, etc. I then began his program.

After a couple weeks, I started to regain some energy, and my BMs lessened through the changes in my diet. Previously, my doctor had explained to me that diet nor stress had anything to do with my UC!! I always found this quite hard to believe. After continuing to improve while working with Greg and following his every direction and some trial and error, I was beginning to get my weight back, was able to work out a bit, and had a huge increase in energy that was beneficial to my overall health as well as interaction with my wife and daughter.

I began to feel so good that I was able to ween off of Humira, and have felt 10 years younger and full of energy since. My programme is about to come to an end, and I have no worries that I cannot continue to feel healthy and energetic. I can enjoy social interaction, go to work related events and enjoy all of my time with my wife and daughter again.

Greg has been absolutely phenomenal!!!! I never thought I could feel half as good as I do now, and I owe such a huge debt of gratitude for his work with my disease. If you have UC or

Crohns and are wondering if it would be a good idea to reach out to Greg, PLEASE DO IT! I have gone from hopeless despair to being as healthy as I can ever remember. Greg, you are AWESOME! Thanks so much" - **Tony Zambrellow**

"I have always tried to live a relatively healthy lifestyle however all ways just seemed to be ill one way or another. After spending years going round in circles with the doctors and hospitals I felt that I was getting nowhere and then when I was diagnosed with Undetermined colitis at 28 I was devastated and led to believe that I would require medication for life. Of course this was the worst thing I could have ever been told, and I was VERY reluctant to take the medications. However, I tried everything they gave me and of course I was right, nothing was helping.

I was then admitted to the hospital and after 9 days told I had Clostridium difficile (C.Diff) on top of the colitis and again pumped with more medication. Quickly after being discharged from hospital I decided I no longer was going to be controlled and restricted by the medication. I knew I had to do something very quickly to try to fix this, and decided that going private was now my only option.

I scrolled the internet for days and by change came across Greg's webinar. When he said that he could help I was extremely sceptical but thought emm I'm interested. So I arranged a call with Greg and then decided to work with him and to be honest at this point I thought what have I done he won't be able to help me! HOW WRONG I WAS! I am very stubborn so admitting I'm wrong is not something I do lightly. However working with Greg has been the best thing I have ever done. Not only have my health and confidence improved and increased but I am still completely medication free and living a much better quality of life.

The process was not at all as bad as I imagined it to be, Greg keeps it very realistic to your lifestyle and is on hand to guide you through it all, and for me being very stubborn I often found that I needed this support and to talk through things in depth before I did them and Greg was never anything but helpful, understanding and supportive throughout.

My advice would be, if you are looking for a manageable and natural way to learn to live with and control symptoms then you have to work with Greg it was the best thing I have ever done and will eternally be grateful for all the help and support he has provided to me through out." - **Louise Sharp**

"I started working with Greg soon after I had been first diagnosed with Crohn's. The medical profession were trying to encourage me to take huge does of steroids. I had seen so many of my patients at work suffer so much, partly due to the side effects of medications they had been given and so was determined that that was not the way I wanted to manage my Crohn's.

I had researched other ways of managing it online but there were so many different diets suggested that to be honest it was all a bit confusing, but I knew there must be a better way than taking a cocktail of drugs with huge side effects. Greg and one of his members of staff Jennifer's help was invaluable as they had a similar ethos and had the knowledge that I didn't and were able to fill in the gaps that I would probably never have worked out.

The whole process was clear and it was so helpful to touch base and process what had been going on for the preceeding few weeks and to have really sensible suggestions that I hadn't thought of. Greg was able to help me in an extremely holistic way looking at so many life-style factors: diet, stress, toxins, all of which have had such a positive impact on my life.

Although I am not completely symptom free all the time, over the period of time working with Greg and Jennifer, I have been able to work out what my particular triggers are (in particular wheat and grains) and the huge impact stress has on my symptoms, this was really noticeable whilst on holiday when I was pretty much symptom free. In day to day life thanks to Greg, I am now able to manage my symptoms and if they do return I am able to work out what has triggered them and get back on top of things.

Without Greg filling in the gaps of my knowledge, I think this would still be an enigma. It was a big investment but I am so thankful that I am able to manage the condition without a cocktail of drugs some with life changing side effects.

When I started work with him, I was exhausted all the time having spent around 10 months not absorbing anything. The idea of going out in the evening was an impossibility.

I am now back to my normal energised self and can pretty much keep up with anything now, working nearly full time, fostering, taxi-ing three teenage girls around and lots of long walks with our lovely Labrador, which is such a contrast to when I started working with Greg 10 months ago when everything was a struggle and I had felt I had to ration where I was going to invest where my energy as there was so little of it." - **Jennie Slatter**

"Before working with Greg I had been suffering with constant diarrhoea, low energy levels, and lack of appetite for many months, caused by ulcerative colitis. I desperately wanted to get my health back and once again enjoy swimming, yoga,

vegetable gardening and cycling. All these activities were impossible as I just felt so weak and exhausted all the time, and was unable to stray very far away from a toilet!

The prescribed ever-increasing medication from the IBD clinic was not helping very much, and if anything seemed to be making matters worse. Disillusioned with hospital GI specialists, strong UC drugs and invasive medical procedures, I started searching the Internet, and Facebook to see what others were doing for their ulcerative colitis. Here I met so many conflicting opinions and advice, some of it was almost laughable and unbelievable, but mostly it was very confusing and depressing. However, what I did learn was that each person is very different and what might work for one would not necessarily help another person with their UC.

What I wanted was a personalised programme based on MY symptoms and what I was eating or unable to eat. Also, I wanted to know exactly what was happening to MY gut and innards that were causing me to be so ill, something my doctors and even the IBD nurses seemed to think was an extraordinary request! But I also wanted help from someone who knew what they were up against, someone who knew precisely what I was experiencing with an ulcerative colitis flare-up, and had a good and proven success rate with their treatment.

Greg seemed the ideal choice to help me, as his wife had suffered badly from ulcerative colitis in the past and he had successfully helped her regain and maintain full health. I was impressed that he could arrange for a comprehensive 3 day stool test which would indicate clearly what my gut was having difficulty with, something no doctor had ever offered or suggested to me!

Initially I was concerned at the costs involved, but decided that I would be making a valuable investment to my future well-

being. To begin with keeping a food diary for several weeks was a bit daunting, but it certainly encouraged me to eat regular proper meals again and be guided into making wiser food choices.

Test results revealed that my gut was in very poor condition. Greg suggested and supplied several supplements for me to take short term, along with my existing medication, to improve and support my gut flora.

Gradually with Greg's guidance, supplements, and food choice suggestions I had a better day now and again, was eating tasty food, and beginning to feel more in control. Good days became more frequent, and my energy levels began to improve, with toilet visits becoming less frequent. Three months into the programme I was feeling much better, good days were outweighing bad days and I was confident enough to start swimming again, returned to yoga classes, and began to take an interest in my neglected vegetable garden once more. I was enjoying a much wider range of food, and learning all the time about healthier eating and how to further improve my eating habits.

My husband had been very concerned with how ill I had been and was relieved to see me regaining my strength and interest in life. We started cycling together again, going walking, and even eating out occasionally.

Towards the end of Greg's programme I felt so healthy and full of energy it was almost unbelievable! Now bad days and constant toilet visits no longer exist for me. I am currently on minimum medication, taking a couple of supplements daily, eating well, bouncing around full of energy, and couldn't be happier with such an amazing turnaround. Life really is good once more! I am so grateful to Greg for all the help and hard work he put into a comprehensive programme to get me well again.

If you are thinking of maybe working with Greg, but are hesitating then I'd say, go on, you're worth it – you have nothing to lose. He is so easy to work with, is very understanding and knowledgeable, and has a great sense of humour. Invest and enjoy the journey back to good health." -
Liz Booker

Thank you for reading. For more success stories then visit <u>www.IamGregWilliams.com</u>

Printed in Great Britain
by Amazon